out of
HIDING

REMOVING THE MASK ⟫→ DAHLIA RODGERS

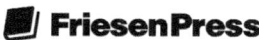

FriesenPress

Suite 300 - 990 Fort St
Victoria, BC, Canada, V8V 3K2
www.friesenpress.com

ISBN
978-1-4602-2470-0 (Hardcover)
978-1-4602-2471-7 (Paperback)
978-1-4602-2472-4 (eBook)

1. Health & Fitness, Diseases, Immune System

Distributed to the trade by The Ingram Book Company

Dahlia Rodgers

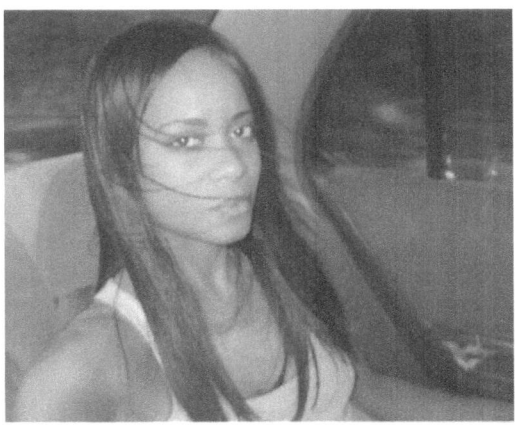

Dahlia Rodgers is a 31 year old female, born and raised in Brooklyn, NY. As a young girl she was very ambitious, confident, determined, fearless and rebellious, causing her to encounter many life obstacles. The bad has out weighed the good, but the Good has served its purposed. Dahlia has grown into a strong, spiritual woman who is not only thankful for her past but also embraces and loves life with all the ups and downs that it comes with. She still resides in Brooklyn, NY, with her 8 year old daughter. She is pursuing a nursing degree at CUNY MEDGAR EVER COLLEGE, Attending church once a week, training in the gym and for the last three years has been the Care taker of her aunt that suffers from Alzheimer's.

Chapter 1

It was Saturday morning. I rolled over on my back, facing the ceiling. I thought about my future. I smiled and said to myself, *When I turn seventeen, I want to have my first child; when I turn eighteen, I want to have my second child. I want to climb these steps until I have been blessed with five children.* I imagined and smiled, convinced I would be the best mommy in the world.

Mom yelled, "Jobe, come and eat your breakfast!"

I jumped out of bed and ran to the kitchen table with all my happy thoughts of having a big family of my own one day.

I'm not sure why, at the age of thirteen, parenting meant so much to me, but it did. I never had a boyfriend, and I was not into liking boys as yet.

Mom cooked pancakes and sausages, along with my favourite: hot chocolate. Even though this was my breakfast, chocolate milk was something that I needed to drink at least three times per day. I drank chocolate milk at any room temperature. My mom would make enough chocolate milk for me that once I arrived home from school, my first stop would be the kitchen, where I would drink the remainder of my chocolate milk. And no, it was not spoiled. Then the next time I needed my chocolate milk was right before bed. My mom would make a cup of fresh chocolate milk for me. It was chocolate powder, sugar, and skim milk mixed together. This went on until I was about eighteen years old. which is around the time I moved into my first apartment.

We lived in a small complex that resembled the projects. The complex was built on a huge tennis court/recreational center. It was broken down, and then they built twenty three-story buildings in the complex. It was a safe place, with a low crime rate and two huge parks on each side of the complex. There were about sixty kids living in the complex. It was a decent place for raising children. Because we never left the complex, Mom was able to look out the window and see us playing. If we went to another building or to the park, that still was not a far distance for her to find us. There were a lot of trees, which brought a lot of life to the place, and most of the different families got along very well.

That day was an exciting day for me. I would be involved in a lot of activities with the boys in the complex. I enjoyed playing with the boys more than I did with the girls. We played baseball, which was my favourite sport. We ran races against each other, and we played red light, green light, 1-2-3. There were always cool activities to play. The girls only jumped rope and played hopscotch. For me, that was boring. Some days I even wished I was a boy. I can now say that the boys' activities were more challenging. Some days, when we felt mischievous, we would have water fights, throw water balloons at people from the top of the roof, or go to the top floor of the building and bang on doors while running to the bottom floor. Sometimes we made it to the bottom floor, and sometimes we ended up in a pile on top of each other because of fighting to get past each other.

The person on the bottom of the pile usually was hurt bad enough that he/she would stay in the hallway crying, and whoever did come out would blame him/her for knocking on their door.

Next, the person would go to that child's apartment and complain to his or her parents. If I ended up on the bottom of the pile, I would scream for everyone to get off of me and in my pain I would get up and continue running until I was outside the building. I would then start crying and beat up whoever felt it was funny. I played fight with the boys all the time. I was like a tomboy, so I was not scared to start a real fight. Some days we would climb the tallest tree and have little chats. We would also get creative and make things. We made a cool go-kart once, and another time we built a clubhouse out of bricks and cardboard.

When I did not have to focus on anything in particular, I spent my time thinking. Most of my favourite thoughts were about having five kids, owning my own business, and being able to take care of my close and extended family. I thought about making my mom the most proud mom in the world. I wanted to accomplish this just as much as I wanted to have my five children. I wished to be able to buy my mom whatever she wanted and travel with her to different places all over the world. I was what you would call an extreme momma's baby. My mom meant the world to me.

My mother was a beautiful, tall, fair-skinned lady, with thick hair that resembled a wig (but it was her natural hair). Her name was Athena.

She was born in the land of paradise: Montego Bay, Jamaica. She came to America at the age of eighteen. By thirty-two, she had given birth to my two sisters and myself. We did not grow up with our father, but my mom's strong personality and dedication to her kids dominated that part of life and made me who I am today. I don't know what it's like to have a father, and sometimes I feel like I missed out. I think that having my father around would have caused me to make better decisions in life: the boys I chose to date, hustling, getting better grades in school, etc. I also think maybe he could have grounded me. Overall, I learned strong independent qualities from my mom.

My mom, my sisters, and myself went from cleaning, to cooking, to taking turns each week to wash three huge loads of laundry by ourselves, to learning how to ride a bike, to patching bicycle tires, to painting the whole apartment together, to changing pipes under the sink, to learing to drive, etc. My favourite lesson, which I'm thankful for today, is how to stay out of credit card debt. Even though I did not grow up with my father, I knew of him and saw him from time to time. When I was about nine years old, my father worked for a driving school. I called the driving school and asked to speak to him.

The female who answered the phone asked me for my name. I responded and said Jobe. I heard when she relayed that message to him; she came back on the phone and said to me that he said he did not know anyone by that name. I then said to her that it was his daughter, Jobe. She let him know that it was his daughter calling, then came back on the phone and said again that he did not know anyone named Jobe. You can imagine how I felt, just nine years old. My heart felt heavy, like someone had placed a house on my tiny chest. I wanted to cry and I couldn't. It scarred me for years. I one day said to myself that I would wait on my father to love me, and when he did, I would forgive him.

In the meantime, I grew to dislike boys and life. When my father did come around, probably every two years, he always had the same thing in his hand. He had a small cooler filled with ice, a 151-proof Devil's Spring bottle of liquor, and a Sprite. My father was tall, handsome, and well-groomed, an elderly man who always claimed to be eighteen years old. I honestly think it was foolish of him to claim eighteen years of age when the legal age for drinking Devil's Spring was twenty-one, but that was his thing. He was born in North Carolina, and I'm not sure how he made it to New York. He would come by and start drinking, then when the liquor kicked in, he spoke mostly about God.

He was a Jehovah's Witness, and my mom was a Christian, He would argue with her as to why her religion and beliefs were wrong until around 12am she would kick him out. That's all I really knew about him. As I grew older, I realized how much of a drunk, arrogant, self-centered, egotistical, deadbeat dad he was, but I still waited for him to love me. This anger stayed with me until my early thirties. I sometimes felt that he ruined my life. The thought of him sometimes made me angry, and I would bully kids at school. Sometimes I even picked fights with the kids in the complex.

One day, there was a pair of blue and white Nike Uptowns out new in stores. The cost of the sneakers was $30. I wanted these sneakers very badly. I asked my mom for the $30 to purchase the sneakers. My mom said no and that she could not afford it. Being the spoiled brat that I was, I cried and begged. My mom then went into her savings and gave me the money. Her savings was always in a coat pocket in her closet. Not much of a savings if it could fit into a coat pocket, but by the grace of God, she worked miracles. I felt bad, even though I should have felt happy.

I pondered and said to myself, *If I find a way to make money to buy the things I want, Mom will be able to save her money and buy the things she wants for herself.* Even though I felt bad, I left and purchased my new sneakers. Back in the day, we didn't really care what our clothes looked like, but our sneakers had to be fly.

Nothing compared to wearing a fresh pair of sneakers. Sometimes when I couldn't afford to purchase my size sneakers, sadly, I would purchase a size three while knowing I was a size four, just to pay the lesser price. The consequences of that were growing two corns on each of my ten toes before I was sixteen. I became so embarrassed with my toes that I never wore open-toed shoes. I always wore socks, and if I did go to the beach or pool, I would isolate myself. Only when I got into the water would I set my toes free.

Chapter 2

It's Monday morning, and Mom yells, "Jobe, get out of bed! Come and eat your breakfast and get ready for school."

I jumped out of bed and ran into the bathroom, my mind occupied with so many thoughts. Yet I was able to function normally. I brushed my teeth and washed my face, then ran to the table. I was always running everywhere I went, no matter the distance. I started running track in high school, and after a bad fall, I decided to quit. I had a passion for running, and I should have felt bad about the decision that I made, but I did not. I was on the track team for about two weeks. I ran my first race on the school's outdoor field. It was a 100 meter race, and I ran against the team's fastest runner. I won the race. I ran past the finish line, then I fell.

I was the type of child who thrived on challenges. I felt that if she was the fastest runner on the team, and it was such an easy win, running was a waste of my time. I would do something else. Today I can only shake my head. I later did go ahead and try out for basketball, , and volleyball, but unfortunately nothing stuck. I wanted to try karate and gymnastics, but those sports were not offered for free at my school, and my mom could not afford to pay for them. I liked to dance, and I was in a dance class. That didn't go too well because of my frequent mood swings.

One day I was nice and engaging, and another day I was distant and antisocial. When we entered dance class, we all would lay our bags and coats on a mat. One day, a girl name Regina did not take part in the dance lesson. She sat alone next to the coats and bags. I'm not sure what attracted her to my coat—it was not fancy, colourful, or brand new, but an old jean jacket I'd had for about two years. Dance class was my last period for the day. I usually saved the quarters my mom gave me for the week until I had $2. My mom would give me fifty cents a day to go to school, therefore it took me four days to save $2. I would then change the coins for two-dollar bills. I was never bothered by this, because It was a treat for me on a Friday to purchase a small box of cheese French fries.

This Friday, I rushed out of class and headed to Wendy's to get my cheese French fries. I opened my coat pocket and noticed that my $2 were missing. My anger kicked in, and I dropped my book bag, took my coat off, and began to search again. Then I stood there, perplexed. I went home angry. For the remainder of the day, I would be okay, and then I would start to think about my $2. I couldn't sleep that night, so I woke up, went into the bathroom, and decided to write a poem.

Tonight I'm sad

Tonight I'm sad,

I went to school and lost all the money that I had,

Why does life have to be so unfair?

All the pain and hurt that I have to bear.

If God would just make me rich,

I would not have to go through this.

Tonight I'm sad and I cry

Because after school I was

Not able to purchase my cheese fries.

I was not a fan of the dark, so after writing I began to panic. The house was dark, and I was the only one up. I was not able to sleep. I decided to leave my sister in bed and go sleep with my mom in the living room. When I tried to get in bed with her, she asked me what I was doing. I told her I was scared, and the cursing that I got from her made my night worse. She yelled at me for waking her up. I wished I had turned on the light first, because she told me to go back to my bed. I asked her to follow me. I felt a blow to my head, and I knew I had to run. I returned to my bed and convinced myself I saw spirits floating in the room. I was scared out of my mind.

I decided I was not going to close my eyes. I'm not sure when I fell asleep, but awoke to a bright Sunday morning. This day was going pretty well until I decided to retrace my steps from Friday to find my $2. I stumbled across an interesting image of Regina sitting next to the coats. I thought then that Regina stole my $2, and I was going to strangle her. I couldn't wait for Friday dance class to arrive. I was so mad that when I saw Regina, I grabbed her and pushed her against the window in the dance class. I knew I didn't have much time to kick her butt before the teacher arrived.

The others kids were happy to see the chaos taking place. Regina asked me what she had done, and I told she had stolen my $2.

Thank God it turned out that she *did* steal it, because I hit her before I found out. She was so scared that she said sorry and she would get the money back from her father and bring it to me the following Friday. I took a book out my bag and told her that if she didn't give me my money back, I was going to use the book to slap her on the back of her head and then I would bring my gang. I did not have a gang, nor was I affiliated with any of the sort, but I noticed how afraid she was—and I wanted my $2 back. By the following Friday I had $4, and I was in heaven.

I finished my breakfast and was anxious to put on my clothing with my new sneakers. It was 8:30am. I ran out the door and straight to school. I never liked to be late only for my first period. For my other classes, I would hang out in the hallway until about five minutes after my class started. My occupied mind made school extremely hard. I would stare at the teacher and not hear a word she said. Nothing ever registered, because I was too busy thinking about other things. If it was a class I didn't like—for example, Global Studies—I would write poems, daydream, draw, or go to sleep. Science was my favourite subject, and I did very well at it. I was not good at math, but it was another favourite subject.

I had my ups and downs in school. Some days I liked it, and some days I didn't, but I always felt good about completing a day of school, which I really did not want to attend. That taught me a lesson: even though I didn't want to do something that had to be done, I had to force myself to do it so I didn't have to repeat it at a later time in life. I knew I wanted my diploma, and I did what I had to do to accomplish that. I wish I wanted my degree just as badly when I started college. I did not want to settle for a GED, and I knew I had to stay in school, attend my classes, and get 65% to pass my class. It was not my best, but it is what was required, and that's what I did. I wanted a Regent's diploma, but I was ok with just passing my RCTs to get my diploma.

I always heard people say that you could go to college even when you were eighty years old. I wish I didn't take that in. That is one of the reasons I never finished when I should have. My major was social work at the time. I finished my internship, and if I'm remembering correctly, I had four classes left to complete my degree. With all of my stress from making money and friends, I dropped out with the assumption that I could return to college at a later time in life and finish. Rebellion, determination, and anger had gotten the best of me. I actually thought I was in control of my destiny and that I had all the answers.

I had to find a way to make money. I was too young to get a job. I had friends in school in my grade and my same age, but I always felt older than them. Their conversations and interests bored me. I kept those thoughts to myself and mingled anyway. They were into boys, gossip, and very girlie things like hair, nails, and makeup. I was moody, and into passing my classes so I could graduate on time, getting the day over with so I could go and make money. I realized that the teacher based our grades on our tests. I made sure I passed all tests, even if I had to cheat. I did what I had to do to graduate, even though I can now say I cheated myself. I did graduate on time, the only one out of five friends.

I remember one day walking in the hallway with my yearbook. One of the security guards took notice and had the audacity to ask if I was really graduating. He was in shock. I told him not to be mad because in high school he hung out in the hallways and got left back. He laughed and shook his head. I rolled my eyes and went on my way.

Chapter 3

I came up with a plan for making money. I went home and showed my mom two of my tests I had honestly passed. One was a science test I had received a 75% grade on, and one was a reading test I had received 82% on. My mom took the test from me, holding both in one hand. She kissed them, thanked the Lord, and handed them back to me. I then asked my mom for one dollar in reward for passing the two tests. She went over to her purse and handed me four quarters. My thought at the moment was, *I will never ask my mom for another penny. My life will change forever.*

On Saturday morning my mom did not have to wake me up. I jumped out of bed at around 8am, ran to the bathroom, brushed my teeth, and washed my face. I told my mom I would have some cereal for breakfast. My mom was a home health aid and exhausted from long hours of work and being paid minimum wage. By the grace of God, she managed to raise three kids. My older sister, my younger sister, and myself. As I ate my cereal, I pondered and smiled. I was determined, motivated, and ready to start making money for myself.

Chapter 4

It was a nice cool day outside, about 55 degrees. I was dressed warm enough to keep me comfortable throughout the day. I had to prepare myself, because I was going to be doing a lot of walking. My mom allowed me to go outside and play until 7pm. I was very responsible, so Mommy didn't always have to watch me. I walked about two blocks to the candy store. I looked through all the boxes of chocolate bars. There was a Snickers box that was almost empty. I purchased two Snickers bars totalling $1. I asked the man at the counter if I could please put the remaining Snickers into another Snickers box and keep one in my hand. The gentleman smiled and said yes. I put my two Snickers bars into the box and left the store.

I walked up to a lady and said, "Good afternoon, ma'am, I am selling chocolate for my cheerleading squad to purchase new uniforms. Would you like to support us by purchasing a Snickers bar for one dollar?" I added, "If you do not wish to purchase a chocolate bar, a donation of anything— including a penny—will be thankful."

The lady smiled and replied, "Sure, I would love to support." She purchased both of the chocolate bars, and I made my first $2. I walked to the nearest candy store and purchased four Snickers bars with the $2 I had just made. I placed them in my box and repeated the process for the next six hours. I was not on a cheerleading team, but I had to say I was selling my chocolate for a good purpose. I knew I had to be home by 7pm, so at around 5pm, I continued to sell, working my way back home.

I pondered on my way back home and decided that I would not tell my mom about my way of making money yet. I made it home at around 7:10pm. Mom was still cooking dinner, and my sisters were in the living room watching television. I threw my box away with intentions of asking for a brand new one the next day. My money was rolled up in my pocket. I went into the bathroom, locked the door, and counted it. After selling chocolate and taking donations, I had made $48 in the first day. I was extremely excited. I felt like screaming, but instead quietly jumped up and down in the bathroom, celebrating. I thought to myself, *I have to find a way to go to school, work after school, and return home by 7pm. I am only in the ninth grade, and school finishes at 3pm. I am more determined to graduate from high school.* I assumed in college I would have shorter hours. I would then have more time to make money.

For the next few months, I was able to sell chocolate and make it home on time. The school year was almost out, and I had saved $840. I convinced myself that I was a businesswoman and gave my chocolate business a name. I called it "Yummy Sports." I kept that name to myself because of all the different sports I was selling chocolate for. The name was just to convince myself that I was running an honest, successful business.

I had to tell my mom. School was out, and I was going to have a great summer, God willing. Then I decided to take a different route to sell my chocolate. I walked for about one hour and came to a street called Erroneous Street, which had a big Terminal Market. I went inside the terminal market, where there were a variety of things being sold. I walked into one of the stores in the Terminal Market, and a guy was selling a variety of chocolate bars by the box. I was in heaven. I purchased a box of 51 M&Ms packages for $17. I also purchased a box of Snickers for the same price. This for me meant more product and more money. I would put one box in my book bag and the other in my hand. I made sure to leave home with enough time that I would be able to sell both boxes and be home by 7pm. I no longer had to go back and forth to the different candy stores to load up.

I knew I had to tell my mom how I was making money, because I would not be able to hide the boxes from her, and she would want to know what I was doing with them and how I got them. This day I was not able to sell both boxes, but I did sell more than one box. By luck, I was able to find the Terminal Market and make it home before 7pm. I made it home at around 6:50pm. I put the remainder of my chocolate in my book bag.

I went into my mom's room and told her that I wanted to speak with her. She asked if everything was okay. I told her yes, that I had found a way to make money and I had saved a little more than $840. My mom's eyes popped out of her head, her forehead wrinkled, and she took a big breath in and out. I spoke again and said I had to pee. She then said, "If you walk out of this room, you will never pee again in your life." I decided that having to pee was not a good idea. My mother then said, "Please explain to me exactly what you have been doing to make money."

In a low voice and sad facial expression, I explained it to her, starting with the day I asked for a pair of sneakers and how bad I felt. I then went into the reason why I asked her for the dollar and how it all started. I concluded my story by letting her know that I just wanted to make her a proud mom. My mom asked me where the money was. I went into my hiding spot (which was in one of my drawers), took the money out, and handed it to her. My mom counted the money and held her head in disbelief. She said, "You want to make me a proud mom by becoming a mini chocolate dealer." She told me that she was not proud, that she was disappointed, and that she did not want me to ever go behind her back and do something like this.

She said it was not safe and she did not approve of it in her house. She said if I wanted to make her a proud mom, it was through school—getting good grades and passing my classes. She added that school was all I needed to be focused on. I thought she was finished, but her pointer finger went up. I braced myself against the door. She pointed her finger in my face and said she was not busting her butt, working double shifts, and taking care of me to get a phone call that something had happened to me on the streets. I agreed with my mom and told her I would not sell chocolate anymore.

My mom then gave me back my $840 and told me that young girls did not belong in the streets. I thought I would wait for things to calm down, then ask my mom to take me to the mall. I wanted a BMX bike, a baseball set, and the new Jordans. The thought that I'd actually made $840 and was now able to buy things for myself was amazing. I started to think about inventing something and getting rich that way.

Chapter 5

Days have gone by, and I think about how much money I could have made. I was an obedient child, but for once I was determined to break the rules. I had a plan. I had a close friend named Yiddish. Yiddish lived in the apartment building behind my own. It was around midday when I went over to her house and rang her bell. Yiddish had the music blasting and as usual she was making up new dance moves. Dancing was something most of the girls in the complex enjoyed doing. We would have dance competitions against each other, or we would all get together in groups and make up different dance routines. I told her to turn off the radio, because I had some good news.

Yiddish immediately became excited, and in her curious voice she said, "Girl, what happened?"

I said that nothing happened, I'd just found a way to make some money and we both could do it and buy new Jordans. Yiddish loved the Jordan sneakers, and this was my way of attempting to pull her in. Yiddish was older than me by two years, but we had been friends for a long time. I explained to her what we had to do, and to make it even more interesting, I even offered to purchase her first two boxes of chocolate to start her off. Of course, she had to reimburse me at the end of the day. Yiddish was very excited, and we both agreed to start selling chocolate together the following day. I was excited because I had someone to go with and somewhere to hide my chocolate if I didn't sell it all.

Mommy liked Yiddish, so whenever I went out to play I would tell my mom that I was going by Yiddish's house or to the park. Yiddish and I sold chocolate almost every day in the summer. I continued to save my money. While selling my chocolate, I was always asked if there was anything to sign. I decided to turn it up a notch by typing a letter stating what school I was attending and what I was supposedly selling the chocolate bars for. I also made a cover letter with girls' cheerleading as a header and really colourful letters, stating that it was a fundraiser. The last page was numbered 1-30 with blank lines. There was a row for your name, your address, and for the donation you were giving. As I walked and sold chocolate, I presented these papers to make it look even more official. Most of the time I saved my money. Yiddish sold her chocolate, and because we would end up near shopping malls or little sneakers stores, she always purchased herself a new pair of sneakers or new clothing.

One day Yiddish called me to let me know that she wanted to go to the nail salon before going to sell chocolate. At the time I was home writing the words to a song called "Shoop" by TLC. I liked that song and wanted to know how to sing along. That was something I did often. I told Yiddish to go ahead and that I would meet her at the nail salon. About an hour later, I left the house and walked to the nail salon. When I saw Yiddish, she was drying her nails. The nails were as long as her fingers and dark blue. I asked her if she would be able to pick up the chocolate bars to sell them with those long nails. She said, "What, you don't like my sexy nails? I thought I would be nice, and I said your claws are cute." She rolled her eyes and said "Whatever, girl, my nails are hot."

I'd never had my nails done, and her nails were the normal fake nail length, but for me they looked abnormally long. For the remainder of the day, Yiddish was no longer Yiddish. She was supposedly L'il Kim, getting on my nerves with her new nails.

Chapter 6

Yiddish and I had grown very close. She was able to shop more than me because she had more freedom. As for me, I would have to answer a million questions. My mom had no clue I was still selling chocolate. Yiddish and I had been walking extremely long distances to sell chocolate. Some days we even rode the trains, travelling to other boroughs we were not familiar with. That's where learning to read the subway map came into play. We tried to get all six boxes of chocolate sold before the day was over. Whoever finished first helped the other person finish selling their chocolate bars, and then we would head home. One day, while selling our chocolate bars in the city, a man that we approached asked us where our IDs were. He stated that he was from the board of ED. He said that when selling chocolate for any event, we were supposed to wear a chain with an ID. We both became nervous and ran off. I was absolutely not going to wear a chain with my ID.

Months had gone by, and we were still selling chocolate. Another day, I went into a record store and approached a man, trying to sell him a Snickers bar. The man looked at me and replied, "You still didn't get your uniforms." He added, "You have been selling chocolate for ten years."

I paused, in shock. I replied, "These uniforms are for a different team." That was the first thing that came to mind. The man said I should come back next week. I thought, *Come back next week to purchase a chocolate bar. What a cheapskate.*

The weekend was approaching, and Yiddish told me about a house party coming up. I was excited and really wanted to go. When I get home, I told my mom about the party and asked her if I could go. She said she had to know the address, and the name and number of the person having the party. Totally embarrassing, but I did want to go. I got all the information from Yiddish and gave it to Mom. Yiddish and I purchased new clothes for the party. Yiddish kept my new clothes at her house. I purchased a nice pair of jeans and a cute fitted shirt. I didn't shop like Yiddish, but making my own money and buying the things I wanted was so cool.

The experience caused me to ponder even more the idea of opening my own business one day. I thought about a discount store, a gas station, or a home for the mentally challenged. I wanted something that was high in demand. I remember us going into a real estate business. After selling chocolate to the lady, I asked her what the cheapest building cost. She said about $300,000. I thought to myself, *That's a lot of chocolate to sell.* When leaving the real estate place, I asked Yiddish if she thought we could make $300,000 selling chocolate. Yiddish laughed and said, "Let's try it."

I said, But where would we save the money?"

Yiddish replied, "At my house, dummy."

I said, No way—you will open your own Jordan shop."

Yiddish laughed and said, "You know, that's kind of true."

I asked Yiddish how much money she had saved already from selling chocolate. Yiddish replied that she always had a lot of things to do, so she had not been able to save, but she was going to start. I said to Yiddish that maybe buying a building was not a great idea after all.

Yiddish changed the topic and talked about the party we were planning to attend.

Chapter 7

It was Saturday, and I was excited about the party that night. I met with Yiddish and we decided to work, even though we had the party to attend later. While working, we talked about how blessed we were to be young and successful. We spoke about being rich and living luxurious lives. I thought about my five kids and huge house.

We then walked into a Chinese restaurant to sell our chocolate. The guy we approached did not want to purchase a chocolate bar, but he did say he would make a $5 donation if we did a Cheerleading step for him. We both looked at each other in shock. We were not on a cheerleading team, and we were far from cheerleaders. What I did instead was turn to Yiddish, and we played a hand game called "Down, down, baby," stomping our feet while doing it. She caught on very quickly. That embarrassing cheerleading session took us about five minutes to finish.

I'm not sure what the man's thoughts were or if he realized that we were not cheerleaders, but he had a huge grin on his face. We smiled as well. I'm not sure if he was smiling with us or at us. He gave us $5 each and told us to stay in school, then left the restaurant. We faced each other and burst out laughing. Yiddish said, "Down, down, baby and cheerleading have nothing in common." I shrugged my shoulders and replied, "It worked."

Today I still practice that philosophy: I would prefer to look foolish for trying than to look foolish for not knowing something that I pretend to know. The most that could come out of such a situation is someone saying, "She is horrible, but at least she's trying."

Yiddish said she actually started to feel like a cheerleader. I told her, "Cheerleaders don't cheer to the Down, down, baby hand game, remember?"

Yiddish laughed and said, "That's because they're not versatile." We both laughed and agreed. The day was dying down, and we made our way back home. Yiddish told me that she'd pick me up at 9pm.

I made it home on time, and Mommy was on the phone. My mom was also in a good mood, She had got a new job working in a nursing home. I was very happy for her. After a few minutes of eavesdropping, I touched her shoulder to get her attention and reminded her that the party was that night and Yiddish was picking me up. She said ok and continued her phone conversation.

I jumped into the shower. Afterwards, I decided to wear my hair gelled and pulled extremely tight into a ponytail. I wore my hair tight so I could have chinky eyes. The things teenagers did for beauty at the time was bittersweet. I threw on something I assumed would look like a party outfit to my mom. By 9pm, Yiddish rang the bell. My mom handed me $10 and told me to be home by 1am. She confirmed all the information that I gave her, I kissed her, then went through the door.

Yiddish and I rushed back to her house for me to change my clothing. Yiddish was an only child, and she lived with her mom. Yiddish's mom worked for a dry cleaner not too far from the block. She gave Yiddish a lot of freedom. Yiddish's mom mostly worked and slept as far as I observed. Yiddish was even in a better school than I was. I guess those are the benefits of being an only child. Yiddish wore pants as well and a top that was very short, exposing her stomach. Her hair was in fine box braids. I was not a party person at the time, but I did love to dance. My favourite music was Reggae and R&B. I was ready to shake a leg until I arrived at the party. There were so many people that I wished I had three boxes of chocolate to sell to everyone. I began to imagine I was standing right at the entrance and stopping everyone before they came in, trying to sell them a chocolate bar. At a certain time, I would walk through the party and sell to anyone else I missed prior to coming to the party. That would absolutely be my type of party.

One of my favourite reggae songs was playing, called "Kun Kum Kum" by Red Dragon. It was a song basically speaking about extremely thin girls. I didn't want to believe I was a Kun Kum Kum, but I was pretty close. I liked the song, and the rhythm was cool as well. I had never danced with a boy before. I did not have anything to drink, because I was underage and thought liquor was absolutely wrong. Instead, I stood in a corner and observed the people and the party. Yiddish was dancing with a guy. She noticed me watching her, stopped, and came over to me. She said, "Why are you not dancing?"

"Because I am relaxing."

Yiddish said I was behaving like I had never been at a party before. She also said I resembled a chinky-eyed plant. I laughed and said, "But plants don't have eyes." I was getting verbally abused for not dancing. I was shy, but I eventually started to sway from right to left. After about thirty minutes, I felt comfortable.

I was very good at dancing, and because I was familiar with the music, it complemented my dance moves. I went off into my own world; it was like it was my birthday party. One of my favourite moves was called the tic-toc. You would basically wind in a circle like a clock ticking. I was enjoying myself. Yiddish left for about ten minutes and returned with a can in her hand. She was drinking beer. She asked me if I wanted a drink. I said no I was fine. She then said that I was dancing like I'd had ten beers. We both laughed, and she joined me. I then realized what dancing looked like after (possibly) one beer. Yiddish was a trip.

I went to use the restroom, and on my way back a guy stopped me and asked me if I wanted to dance. He looked young like me, and I assumed he was my age. I told him to wait. I went over to Yiddish and told her a boy had asked me to dance. I asked her if she thought I should dance with him. I'm not sure why I asked, but she burst out laughing and said, "No, let him dance with you." Guess I deserved that from Yiddish. I walked back to the boy, and we started to dance. I felt mixed emotions dancing with this boy. I felt nervous, but at the same time excited about my first time dancing with a boy. Then slow music came on. I was clueless about the songs being played, and it was obvious I couldn't slow dance. I didn't even bother to try. Instead, I stepped from side to side until he got the picture. He finally decided to take a bathroom break.

Time was going by, and I had to be home for 1am. I went over to Yiddish and told her that the time was now 12:40pm and we should leave. She said okay, and I went back over to the boy I was dancing with and let him know that I was leaving. He asked me what my name was. I told him it was Jobe and he said, "Nice name." I then asked him for his name. "Prudence."

He asked me for my number. I did not own a beeper, and I was not allowed to have boys call the house. I told him he could give me his number and I would call him. He wrote his number on a piece of paper and kissed me on the cheek. I should have been extremely upset, but I was not. I felt mature, I felt high, and I liked it. I thought about my first kiss all the way home. Yiddish and I took a cab home. While in the cab, we spoke about how much fun we'd had and made fun of each other's dance moves. We were totally focused on the wrong thing.

I did not make it home for 1 am. I made it home at around 1:30am and in different clothing. My mom was wide awake and very upset. She yelled at me for coming home late, and then she noticed the different clothing. She then went for my ponytail. I wish I had a quick reflex, allowing me to pull the clip out of my hair before she got to it. She told me to forget about going to another party for the rest of my life. I should have been very upset, but all I could think about was my first kiss and possible first boyfriend, Prudence.

The following day I phoned Yiddish and let her know how much trouble I was in. I told her that we forgot to change my clothing. She laughed and stated that *I* forgot to change my clothing, not *we*. She added, "*You* were rushing to get home." I told her my mom had said that I could not go out for the rest of my life.

Yiddish asked if my mom slept at nights. I said, "Of course she sleeps at night."

Yiddish said, "Great, and I know your windows can open, so you will surely party again." Yiddish added, "And I promise you, when you turn eighteen, you will definitely get to party." She joked about everything, even when she was in trouble.

My mom was on the phone with my aunt, complaining about me coming home late. In her Jamaican accent, she explained how she had grabbed my ponytail. It was going to be a long day. I decided to stay in my room and relax. I didn't bother to tell Yiddish about my possible new boyfriend or my first kiss, because I knew I would never hear the end of the jokes from her, plus I wanted to keep it a secret between me, myself, and I.

Chapter 8

I was fifteen years old, and it had been more than a year since I began dating Prudence. Prudence was a little taller than me. He was very dark-skinned and thin-framed. He was four years older than me. We had a good relationship. I remember going on our first date to a seafood restaurant. We ordered shrimp and lobster. I was allergic, and unable to peel shrimp with my bare hands, so I ate the cooked shrimp. I figured it would be okay. While enjoying my shrimp, my eye started to itch. I used my hand to scratch my eye, and it began to turn red. My eye became very swollen and could not remain open. We had to end our date and go home. Today I still can't eat shrimp. I get a very bad allergic reaction from eating shrimp. Prudence and I also enjoy watching movies together.

Prudence lived in what was called the ghetto, but the brownstone houses were very nice and big. His mom owned a brownstone, and there Prudence lived with his older brother and sister, his nephew, and a younger sister. Prudence had his own room. I would tell my mom that I was going to an afterschool program until 5:30pm every day. That was my way to spend time with Prudence.

Besides watching movies, we enjoyed making mixed tapes and listening to music. I hadn't stopped selling my chocolate, but since I had been dating Prudence, I didn't sell as often. Yiddish and I were not selling chocolate together anymore. She had run into some new friends and was into shoplifting and scamming. I sold with other friends from the complex.

I learned a lot by selling chocolate, and there is one lesson I would like to share. This lesson always played out exactly how I believe it was suppose to. It was like the Lord was teaching me something. It started during the time when Yiddish and I were selling chocolate together. I was selling one day to purchase a new pair of FILA sneakers that had caught my eye.

I made my first $7. Yiddish wanted the same sneakers, so this day was a race between us to get our boxes finished first. Yiddish walked ahead of me at the time, selling her chocolate. She passed the homeless man lying on the pavement. I stopped and, not thinking twice, I handed him the $7 I'd made so far for the morning. It happened so fast. I walked off and thought to myself, *It's cool—I will make my sneaker money.* That day I sold my three boxes of chocolate so fast I thought I was a millionaire.

The money came so quickly, and the donations were $5, $6... a man driving a garbage truck even gave me a $20 donation. Yiddish was upset. She was not having a great day like I was. We had random arguments. She said I had stolen her customer. She would try to run up to people before me. And so on. Anyhow, I did help her finish her boxes. She still was upset at the amount of money I'd made, at me finishing my boxes so fast, and especially at my $20 donation. After selling the three boxes of chocolate, we usually went home with about $160. This day I made almost $200. While walking I started to think. It was like a light turned on in my head.

I envisioned the homeless man lying on the street and giving him $7. I realized that was why I had been so blessed throughout the day. It was because I helped him, truly and from my heart. I helped a stranger that I did not have to help and that I did not know. I obeyed the Lord's order. From that day on, I learned how important it was to help others and that the Lord blesses you to be a blessing to others.

People always said—including Yiddish—that the homeless man could go and get a job, or that he was not really homeless. I would say I didn't know what he was, but for him to be lying on the side of the pavement in a soiled condition… I was most definitely going to help him. I practiced that while selling my chocolate, and I realized that I was not only doing it for me to be blessed, but for the feeling it came with. Helping someone for no apparent reason made me feel amazing. That lesson I carried with me throughout my life.

Today I'm not attached to anything, because I know the value of having nothing but having everything that is priceless. I say this because when you have money, a house, cars, sneakers, success, etc., you tend to feel like you have it all. That is the value of nothing. I don't mean that in a bad way, unless you don't understand your source. Your source is where it all came from. For some people the source is their company, for some it is the boss, for some it is their successful business, etc. My source is the Lord. A company can fail, your boss can fail you, your successful business can fail, but the Lord will never fail you. If you lose all those things, your faith will be tested. Some people rob, steal, commit suicide, or find them-selves doing things they never envisioned themselves doing.

Then you have the people who try to achieve those things. Some try to achieve them honestly, and some do it illegally. In the end, they are discouraged, disappointed, and angry for trying so hard and not accomplishing their goals. When you have everything, that is priceless. Hanging from a tree limb… you are certain you will be ok. You are more at peace with yourself, and you have faith, wisdom, and understanding. You're not worried about tomorrow;

you're thankful when tomorrow comes. Even at your worst, you're confident enough to know you're at your best. You understand that what is for you will be for you, even if it happens before your last breath of air. In that case, you should be able to live without fear and embrace faith. I always tell people that I'm gone with the wind and wherever it takes me, for I am not in control of my destiny, and that is ok. I love to say *Watch my God work*.

My mom and I were arguing a lot back then, and she eventually found out that I was still selling chocolate. She was totally against it. The rebellious child that I had become meant that I'd learned things the hard way. It got to a point where people were makings donations instead of actually purchasing the chocolate bars. I decided to change schools on my head letter and ask for donations to purchase uniforms for the girls' basketball team. I made more money that way, and I did not have to carry the heavy boxes of chocolate anymore. By the time I was completely done asking for donations, I had been on a cheerleading team, a basketball team, a volleyball team, a soccer team, and a track team. I consistently changed my head letter, until one day I decided to get my first real job.

I worked as a cashier in a supermarket. Beforehand, the owner asked me if I would like to get paid on or off the books. I told him off the books. I also had my tip cup at my register. I spoke to the customers and packed their bags very well. I made about $75 in tips by the end of the week. I was paid $250 weekly, plus $75 in tips, and I was okay with that. The owner called me into his office about one month later and told me I could no longer accept tips. He said tips were for other people who wanted to come in and pack bags as a job. I let him know that there was no one there packing bags at any of the registers. I asked if I could accept tips until someone did come. He said no, and I quietly said that it was time to go. I was making more money selling chocolate and asking for donations than what I was making there. I was just settling, because I wanted to make an honest living. I quit that job after a full week of work. I did return for my last paycheck.

One day I woke up not feeling too well. My breast hurt, and I was more tired than normal. I went to school, and my mood was very low. I kept to myself. I looked through the window, and my thoughts started to flow. Instead of listening to the lesson being taught, I decided to write a poem.

My Future . 07-23-2005
Sometimes I sit down in my class,
I look through the window at the green leaves, which remind me of grass.
I look at the trees, I look at the people,
I look at the whole environment, which reminds me of the past,
But that's okay, because the past doesn't last.
I look into the sky,
I think about my future; it feels like it's so close to me,
Only I wish it was a big bright light or picture so I could see.
Sometimes I wonder how my future is going to be,
How I would look or if I would know how to cook.
Or if I would finish college and open a big business,
Or have my own house or even a car,
Or even marry someone I love with two kids and more.
Now I know what I have to do,
Just be successful and true,
Like going to school and not playing the fool,
I know it will work as long as I try hard and stick with God.

I loved to write my thoughts down from time to time. It always made me feel great afterwards.

Prudence was already in high school, and he worked at a super-market stocking boxes. The school day was over, and I was on my way to Prudence's home. When I arrived, he was cleaning his room. I told him how I was feeling, and he asked if my period had come for the month. I didn't keep up with my period, so I was not sure when it was supposed to come. After thinking about it for a few minutes, I realized that it had not come for the month. Prudence got dressed, and we went to the discount store and purchased a pregnancy test. I was embarrassed to be seen purchasing a pregnancy test, so I let him go into the store by himself. At fifteen, I was not comfortable purchasing a pregnancy test, condoms, or sanitary napkins. I totally feared the wrong things. We made our way back to his house.

When we arrived at his home, his mother and older sister greeted us at the door. We hugged and exchanged a few words, then went into his room. We opened the pregnancy test and read the directions. He told me to pee on the strip and cover it afterwards. He kept the box in his room, because he did not want his mom or sister to find it. I went into the bathroom, peed on the strip, and covered it. I returned to the room after washing my hands. By the time I got to the room, there were two pink lines. My pregnancy test was positive. Prudence and I were very happy. We spoke about what the baby might look like, and whether the baby would be a girl or a boy. We spoke about Prudence even getting another job. He was very supportive from the beginning to the end. I had to figure out a way to tell my mom.

I had a huge dream of starting my own family one day, but not at the age of fifteen. Today I can only assume and thank God that things played out the way they did. Not only because they made me who I am today, but because if I had experienced these things at the destined age to start my family, possibly around twenty-three or twenty-four, it would have been harder for me to deal with. When I was younger I was fearless, more of a risk-taker. I did what I felt was right without even thinking twice. When you're young, you're not as alert as you are when you're older. This explains why I was not afraid of becoming a mom. I can also admit that my thoughts on raising a child basically concerned dressing the child in cute clothing, not understanding the bigger responsibilities raising a child came with. This caused me to believe that it was a life-changing decision I could handle. After my first miscarriage, it was a fight that I was determined to win. My faith, determination, and strength prevailed, causing me to become blinded to how young I was. I wanted to win the fight. I was determined to try again. I was going to do whatever it took to bring a baby to term. I told myself if I was not able to accomplish that, then I was not normal and not a worthy human being.

One day I went to the supermarket with my mom. On our way home, I told her I needed to tell her something. She said, "What is it now?" I started to cry and told her I was pregnant. My mom screamed and yelled until we arrived home. My mom had never met Prudence, and I'm not sure she was even aware that I was having sex. I felt completely crushed. By the time we arrived home, my mom calmed down and began asking me the who, what, where, and why. She looked like she wanted to cry. We really didn't speak for more than about thirty minutes. She seemed to be handling the news well, eventually becoming silent and going into the kitchen to cook.

Days went by, and I decided to buy my mom a sorry card to tell her that I was sorry and did not mean to hurt her. She told me that as time went by, it would get better. She added that everything would be okay.

Prudence was keeping up with me and making sure I was okay. He even told all his friends. I didn't tell any of my friends. I was very secretive at the time, and I was not comfortable with any of my friends knowing. I always had a vivid imagination, and I conversed with myself so much that I never felt the need to tell my friends my secrets or thoughts. I would just speak to myself out loud or quietly.

One day I was in my step aerobics class. I participated as if it was a regular day for me, and I was not careful at all. At the age of fifteen, I really didn't know better. After about ten minutes of working out, I decided to sit down. I suddenly felt like my period had come. I asked my teacher if I could please go to the bathroom. I went to the bathroom, and my underwear had blood in it. I thought to myself, *I wonder if I'm bleeding because of all the step climbing.* I rolled up some tissue and placed it in the crotch of my underwear, then went back to class. I told the teacher I did not feel well and asked if it was okay to sit out the remainder of the class. Miss Tiny said, "Sure, Jobe."

After ten minutes, the bell rang and class was over. I was in junior high school, and it was my seventh period class, so I was able to leave school without being stopped by the security guards. I left and went straight to the hospital.

The hospital that I went to was close to my school. It was called Marina Medical Center. When I arrived at the hospital, I went straight to the emergency room. I signed my name on a paper and said what my problem was. This hospital was not very big. It was very crowded, and everyone seemed uneasy after waiting long hours to be seen by a doctor. There was a sign stating that they would see patients according to the severity of their problems.

A lady argued with a man because he'd stepped on her foot. She shouted that he was rude and should have said excuse me and waited for her to move her foot out of the way. He argued back that she should not have had her foot in the way where people had to walk. She said, "It's a free country" and he couldn't tell her what to do. They went back and forth until security came. The yelling got louder, but they eventually stopped when the security officer let them know that they would have to leave the hospital if the arguing continued.

After a while, I decided to go the restroom. My bleeding had stopped, but I was still worried. After about an hour and a half of waiting, my name was called. The doctors took my blood pressure, my weight, and a urine sample. They asked a few questions, then they did a sonogram. I was six weeks pregnant. The doctor spoke peacefully, allowing me to relax. She let me know everything she was doing and what was going on with my baby. The doctor looked for the baby's heartbeat, then informed me that everything was okay. She said that some woman had spots during their pregnancy. She said that if I started to bleed again to come back to the hospital. I was sent home and told to go on bedrest for the remainder of the day.

I was very happy to hear all the good news. When I got home, I called Prudence and updated him on my day. My mom was not home from work. I decided to take a shower and jump into bed. I put on a pad for the spotting. About two hours later, the bleeding started again, and this time it was more heavy. I went to use the bathroom and it looked like running water. I called Prudence immediately, and he rushed over to my home, which was about a twenty-minute drive. He rushed me to the hospital. By the time I got to the hospital, I had soaked the two pads I had on and the inside of my pants. I was seen immediately by a doctor.

The bleeding did not stop. I was crying, lost and confused as to what was going on. I had been to the doctor earlier and everything had been okay. The doctors did another sonogram. They informed me that I was miscarrying. My world tumbled down. I wanted to know why, but they could not tell me much. They said that they could not give me an actual reason why. One of the nurses gave me the famous speech after everything was over. Briefly, that speech was: *You're young, you have your whole life ahead of you. You can always try again later in life,* and on and on. Hearing those words made me feel even worse. They put me to sleep, took out the remainder of what was inside, and cleaned me up. I was given antibiotics to prevent infection, and a small pink pill to stop the bleeding. I was then sent home after I urinated.

Chapter 9

Prudence was very disappointed. He actually made me feel worse than I already did. He said that losing the baby was my fault because I should not have participated in step aerobics. I'd thought to myself that either I participated, or I let the teacher know I was pregnant, which I was not going to do. Hurt, I agreed with him. I started to feel like it was my fault. Prudence didn't know how hurt I was, because I didn't cry while speaking to him. I was embarrassed at what I had done. I developed a slight hate towards myself.

When I arrived home, my mom was lying on the couch. I told her that I had been with the doctor and that I had miscarried. I played tough. I didn't cry while speaking to her. I was too embarrassed. I didn't even tell her that I was doing step aerobics in school. I just told her that I'd started to bleed and had called Prudence. Mom did seem sympathetic, but I knew it was not her dream for me. To comfort her, I told her that I was ok and not ready for a child anyway. While saying that to her, my stomach tightened up, and I feel like I was about to vomit. In reality, I wanted my child and I wished I was still pregnant. My mom then gave me the same famous speech as the nurse had. *You're young, you have your whole life ahead of you, blah blah.*

I went to take a shower, and afterwards Mom gave me some dinner to eat, but I had no appetite. Staring at the plate of food, my emotions started to run, and anger and hurt built up. I wanted to break my spoon in half. Instead, I went to bed. While lying in bed, my mom came into my room and looked at me, then closed the door. I'm sure she knew why I was not able to eat my food. I put my headphones on and listened to music until I fell asleep. I woke up around 2am. I finally opened my eyes. Reality had definitely hit me. I was no longer pregnant, I had killed my baby, and I had disappointed Prudence. I was irresponsible.

I got out of bed and took a sheet of paper and pen from my school bag. I went into the bathroom and closed the door. I started to write a poem.

Life

Life is hard, I wonder why
Life is a struggle and it makes me cry,
Sometimes I sit, and wonder why?
Why did I come in this world and have to die?
I wish there was someone who could answer,
All the questions I wanted to ask,
But I learned it the hard way,
Now it happened to me all in the past.
Someone to teach me to be strong,
Someone to listen just five minutes long,
I'm going through a war where I have to fight,
I'm going to sorrow where there is no light,
I'm going through a pain which is hard to bear,
I've been through a situation which was not fair.
I'm going through a light that is very bright,
I'll hold my head up and keep on trying.
I'll prove what I can do and what I can see,

The most thing I'll prove is that I know I will
And can be all that I can be.

I thought to myself, *I will get pregnant again, and when I do I will do everything different.* I was told by the doctors that as long as I had my Medicaid card and ID, they could see me anytime. That meant I did not need my mom to be with me. With the strong, intelligent, and caring mother that I had, I should have turned to her. Instead I turned to the little voice in my head. Today I thank God for the prayerful and faithful mother I had and that I still have. I may not have turned to her, but I'm sure her prayers played a huge part in me being where I am today. I could have been in my grave, in jail, mentally or physically hurt, and I'm none of these things. While the Lord walked beside me, the Lord was not only moulding me, he was answering my mommy's prayers.

Chapter 10

Days went by, and Prudence and I had been speaking and working on getting things back to normal between us. I started to research how long you should wait to get pregnant again after one miscarriage. I learned that after one to two normal periods, it was okay to try again. I was on a mission. About three weeks after the miscarriage, Prudence gave me a number to call. It was the number for an adolescent center. He said I should start seeing a gynaecologist to make sure everything was okay with me so that I would not miscarry again. I called the number the next day and made an appointment. I was told to bring my school ID and Medicaid card. My appointment was set for five days later. I had never experienced having a GYN, done and I didn't know what to expect, but I was very anxious to get it done. I wanted Prudence to accompany me, but he had to work, so I went by myself. For the next few days, I decided to go online and research GYNs and miscarriages. I watched YouTube videos to see what it was all about. My thoughts were not too good. The procedure looked painful and gross. I closed my eyes and spoke to myself. I said *If you want to have a baby, this is a step that you will have to take to accomplish*. Of course, today I laugh to myself and say it really was not that serious. Also, baby pain was way more painful than having a GYN, yet a GYN checkup scared me more.

That morning I had to take the train uptown to the last stop. I was headed to the adolescent center. When I arrived, they had me sign in. I then filled out some paperwork and remained seated until my name was called. The adolescent center seemed very dull. It was not welcoming, and everything was so closed in and tight. There were a few offices, and of course the exam rooms, with a bunch of teenagers coming in and out. Some of the teenagers were pregnant, with huge tummies.

One female I met told me she was five months pregnant and wanted to have an abortion because her boyfriend broke up with her and did not want the baby. She added that no hospital would do an abortion at five months, so she was coming to the center for counselling for her depression. I felt so bad and confused as to why she would want to kill her baby because of a boy. I wished I was five months pregnant. After about one hour, my name was called. I first saw a social worker, who asked me to fill out a five-page booklet. After completing the booklet, I realized it was a depression test. I'm not sure how I did, but she did go on to ask me questions, mostly about friends and family. After speaking with her, she told me to go into an exam room.

To get a GYN done took about ten minutes. I was happy to experience my first GYN. It was very uncomfortable, but I felt happy about taking care of myself. I was also given an STD test each time I went. They told me that if they didn't call me, my results were fine. I gave them Prudence's cellphone number. I never received a call after my GYN, so I figured I was on my way and prepared to get pregnant again. Six months later, I got my second GYN done and received a call. The doctor explained that they had to do something called a biopsy. The results from the biopsy caused me to have a leep sugery done. He said there were cells that could become cancerous, and they had to cut them out. They then monitored me for one year to make sure the cells did not return.

It did not stop me from getting pregnant a second time. About eight months after my miscarriage, I got pregnant again. At this point, after a miscarriage, a biopsy, and a leep surgery, the hospital would become my second home. I'd tried very hard to get pregnant in the prior months. Every month that I got a negative test, I would feel extremely sad. Getting pregnant and making money were my main interests. I came to the conclusion that working was a waste of time and that making my own money was much better.

A group of five girls from the complex came over to my home. We decided to go on the computer and make sponsor papers. We worked together almost every day. If a new sneaker came out, we would all hustle that amount and we would all purchase the same sneakers. There were five girls—sometimes six—that hustled together. We even formed a dance group called Tantalizing Winners. We would compete in a dancehall queen competition once a month. It was a cool activity that most of the kids in the community looked forward to. We all actually loved to dance. The most interesting part about making up a dance routine was the stunts. We always came up with some awesome stunts. We danced mostly to reggae music. I never spoke about my pregnancy or mis-carriage with any of my friends. That I kept to myself.

One day, I was home, lying on the floor. I felt a tight strain in my vagina. It probably lasted for about two seconds. About a week later, I was on the road hustlingwith my three friends. I let them know that I had to use the restroom. We decided to go into McDonald's to use the restroom, and I noticed a very white thick discharge in my underwear resembling mashed potatoes. I cleaned myself up and told my friends that my menstrual cycle had started and it was best that we made our way home. Most days when I arrived home I would sleep all day, and my breasts were growing slowing. This experience I indirectly paid attention to. It allowed me to learn my body.

I always waited for the end of the first week of a new month to test myself. It was Friday, and I left school and went by Prudence's house. I took my pregnancy test, and sure enough I was pregnant. We were both excited all over again. We decided that we were not going to tell anyone. I hoped Prudence didn't tell anyone, because I was embarrassed about my past miscarriage. Some of his close friends and girlfriends were pregnant, and they were not having any problems. They were either about to give birth or in the nine-month process. I was embarrassed. I decided to go to the doctor right away.

I went to sign up at a different hospital this time for my prenatal care. I went to a hospital called Seaview Hospital This hospital was very big, clean, and welcoming. Being there made me feel like I was not going to have any more complications with my pregnancy. The doctors and nurses were very organized, and I did not have a long wait before I was seen. While waiting for my name to be called, I had thoughts about being pregnant at a young age. Even though having my first child was my desire, I had mixed emotions, one of which was embarrassment. I did not want anyone to know that I was pregnant.

Sometimes when I even spoke to the doctors I felt embarrassed because I was so young and I was pregnant. When they called my name, it was for a procedure like I'd experienced during my last pregnancy. They did a urine test, they took my blood pressure, and then they did a sonogram. Once my pregnancy was confirmed, I was giving a prescription for prenatal pills and iron pills. I was living my days very secretly. After school I would go by Prudence's to sleep. My mom thought I was at after-school. I would eat as much as possible, and I tried to be very careful with everything I did during the day. Just like the first pregnancy, I started to spot at six weeks. By the eighth week it would be more like a light period. I bled every day. I returned to the doctor twice within two weeks, and I was told to go on bedrest. When I sat down, I should sit with my feet up. I was even shown the baby's heartbeat. I figured everything would be ok if there was a heartbeat.

I had very little knowledge about pregnancy. I tried to stay positive during the day. I tried to go to school and work on some days as opposed to everyday. I followed directions as much as possible. At ten weeks pregnant, my world came tumbling down once again. Thank God it was a Friday afternoon when the bleeding started more heavily than normal. I was at Prudence's home at the time. He rushed me to the hospital. They placed me on a stretcher and gave me drops. I felt weak and dizzy. I bled a lot lying there. They finally took me in and did a sonogram. They let me know I was miscarrying.

They said there was a blood clot surrounding the baby. I had no clue at the time what that meant. Today I'm so disturbed by the thought of them giving me an epidural, that I remember it as if it was yesterday. When I woke up, just like the first time, I was giving medication and sent home. I remember seeing the medical doctor before leaving the hospital. I asked her why I had miscarried. She looked at me and responded that usually when a woman miscarried in the first trimester it was because the baby was not developing right. She added that I was young and had my whole life ahead of me. She said I had more than enough time to have a baby. I did not want to hear any of that.

Prudence was disappointed once again. He didn't directly blame me this time. I told him the doctors said it was possibly because the baby was not developing right. He hugged me and said I had done everything right. While walking out of the hospital, I felt a severe pain in my lower back, causing me to lie on the floor in front of the hospital. The pain was so severe that I could not walk. Today I assume it was because of the epidural that was given to me. Prudence was going to call for help, but I didn't want him to let me go. I was in too much pain.

After about ten minutes I told him I had to be home soon and that I couldn't go back into the hospital because my mom might find out that I was pregnant again. I was finally able to get up with his help, and he walked with me slowly to his car. The pain started again, so I decided to go to his house. I could not go home in that position. When we arrived at his home, we met his brother outside.

The pain started again, and silent tears rolled down my face. I wanted to scream, but the slightest movement hurt. I bore the pain until I was once again lying on the ground in front of Prudence's home. Prudence's brother arrived in the middle of everything and asked Prudence what was wrong with me. Prudence told him I'd had a second miscarriage. Prudence's brother argued that I was too young to be going through this and that Prudence was wrong. I was crying and in so much pain, but I refused to go back to the doctor.

Prudence and his brother helped me inside the house. I then had Prudence call my mom, and I told her I was at his house. I did that just to let her know where I was so she would not worry about me. I fell asleep for a few hours. When I woke up, the pain had eased up a lot. I called my mom and told her I was not coming home for the night. I told her I was staying at Prudence's house. She did not agree with me because I was only sixteen at the time, but I was scared to go home and have the pain possibly come back. Prudence was very supportive. He helped me take a shower, gave me some dinner, and we chatted a little bit then watched a movie.

Chapter 11

I was seventeen years old, and life for me was just okay. After my last miscarriage, I decided to give my body a break. I was more determined to have a baby, but I had also been researching miscarriages and staying healthy. On a scale from 1-10, my happiness was at about a 6. Thoughts of not being able to have a child invaded my head daily. Prudence and I were still together, but things had changed as well. He was older than me and he wanted a child very badly, and I might not be able to give him that. With the pain in my heart from my two lost, I still managed to carry on with my life. I was almost done with high school. I had one more year left, and I had a job working in a fast food restaurant named Big Burger. I had stopped selling chocolate and sponsoring completely.

Prudence had started college and worked in a barber shop. Because of having two miscarriages, my number one interest in life was to have a baby. One day I went in to work early, changed my clothes, and headed upstairs to start cashing. The day was going pretty well; my customer service was great, and I even did a little extra work for no apparent reason. About one hour before my clock-out time I went to use the restroom. On my underwear was the same thick white discharge I'd had on my underwear in my last pregnancy. I was puzzled. After I left work, I went and purchased a pregnancy test. By this time I was older and not afraid to purchase a pregnancy test. I went to a Wendy's close to where I worked and took the pregnancy test. My pregnancy test came out positive.

I went to see Prudence and I told him. He was excited, but not as excited as he had been in the past. That was totally understandable. Anyhow, I was excited. I signed up with a different hospital for my prenatal care. I always felt that a different doctor would help me better. I informed the doctors that I'd had two miscarriages. They of course looked at me and asked my age and a lot of other annoying questions at the time. For example: *Are you trying to have a baby? Why are you trying to have a baby? Are you in school?* I knew exactly what they were thinking; however, how I was feeling and what I was going through was all that mattered to me at the time.

Once again I was back to taking my meds, eating right, and trying to become a parent. I was able to sleep over at Prudence's house and my mom was okay with it, she just always wanted me to let her know where I was. We spent a lot of time together during this pregnancy. This time I was considered high risk, which meant bedrest for me during the remainder of the pregnancy. The spotting started at seven weeks. One day I was home, and because of my prior two miscarriages, I knew I was about to miscarry. I went to use the bathroom and urinated; it was mixed with blood and flowed like running water. I felt something like a ball pass as well. I called Prudence, and he rushed over to my home.

My mom was at work still. My sisters were in the living room with their friends. I'm sure they assumed Prudence was just coming to pick me up. I went to the hospital and told the doctors that I believed I was having a miscarriage. The doctors did the usual sonogram, and once again there were blood clots surrounding the baby. The doctors could not explain to me why blood clots surrounded the baby or why I was consistently miscarrying. I was angry with the doctors, myself, and the world.

Chapter 12

Depression had definitely become a part of my life. I felt like I was not human. The Lord made me a female, and I was not able to reproduce.

I would never know what it was like to be a mom. I felt worthless every day of my life. I was quiet, angry, and careless. I gave up selling chocolate and turned to shoplifting. Every day I shoplifted beautiful clothes to dress up with and to feel good about myself. The euphoria I got from getting out of the stores with my new clothing felt great. That's where I found happiness. Jail didn't even scare me. I managed to never do jail time, I always had my bail money or money to pay the police officers off. The most time I ever spent in jail was two days for shoplifting, and afterwards I always went home, took a shower, and if it was early enough, I went right back into the stores.

I shoplifted seven days a week. I had so many clothes and so many things that I did not even need. I'm not even a materialistic person, so most of the things meant nothing to me. Eventually I gave things away to make room for more things. My shoplifting got so bad that I would shoplift things that I *could* afford, even food to eat. I received food stamps to purchase my groceries, but instead I wore a book bag to the supermarket and stole my groceries. I would make about three trips to the car. I know the supermarket didn't have cameras, so it was easy for me to do. As time went by, I learned so much about the stores: how to tell the real from the fake cameras, the blind spots, the alarm systems, how to get off all the different sensors, and last but not least, how to make the workers and undercovers complement my shoplifting behaviour.

I always felt like it was a game we were playing when I saw them. In my mind at the time, I always said they were horrible workers who had no clue how to catch a shoplifter. Some days I would pretend to be hiding or trying to get away from them just so they could follow me everywhere I went in the store. After a few minutes, they would realize what I was doing and walk off. I would follow them everywhere they went in the store. When I realized they were very uncomfortable, I would stop and go steal whatever I wanted. It was so funny to me at the time.

My relationship with Prudence was not going well. He had changed a lot. He was sleeping around, partying and drinking all the time. He even went so far as to tell me that I couldn't have kids. We no longer spent much time together. Prudence said he was busy. Valentine's Day came, and he stopped by my home and gave me a sterling silver bracelet. Then he left. Usually we would go to dinner and the movies, but things had changed. One day I decided to go by Prudence's house. When he went into the shower, I decided to search his phone. I noticed a female named Jezebel consistently coming up. I wrote the number on a piece of paper and decided I would call the next day.

I called around 4pm the next evening. The phone rang, and finally a female answered. I asked if it was Jezebel, and she said yes. I asked her if she knew Prudence. She then asked me if I was his girlfriend. I said yes. She stated that he had been coming to see her for the last four months. She said he'd told her that we were no longer together. This was my first relationship, and I was very inexperienced. I never thought Prudence would cheat on me. I was completely crushed. I asked her if they had slept together, and she said yes. I asked her if she was pregnant. She told me that she was not sure.

Jezebel was Prudence's ex-girlfriend, who he'd been with prior to me and him dating. When he realized that I was not able to have kids, he made up with her and was trying to get her pregnant. I finally phoned Prudence and told him that I'd spoke to Jezebel. I told him I'd got her number out of his phone. Prudence was very upset and specifically told me that I should have never called her, and he said that our relationship was over. He said that I was immature for calling her and that she was who he loved and they'd never really broken up. I was even more heartbroken. My appetite had changed and I looked sickly thin. I totally hated my life. Thoughts of her giving him, my first love, a baby completely crushed me daily.

For some reason, I did not feel the need to put up a fight for our relationship. I took my hurt, because he specifically stated that he did not want to be with me. I thought, *I cannot make someone want to be with me.* I decided to respect his wishes and leave him alone. My days get worse. I couldn't sleep at night, so I stayed up and wrote.

Chapter 13

It was 1999, and I was finally graduating from high school. I was eighteen years old. I did not want to go straight to college. I wanted to get my hair dressing license to have a trade. Once I was finished with hair school, I would pursue a degree in social work and use my trade for income. I decided to research hair schools, and I found one for $9000. Of course I could not afford it, so I decided to give up on that idea. I went on to college and was actually doing very well. My first year, I managed to get a 3.30 GPA. My life consisted of researching miscarriages, shoplifting, and school. I was very depressed, but still able to handle my business, thank God. I can now say that it's sad how a young girl with her whole life ahead of her and endless opportunities was ruined because of wanting and thinking about something that was not necessary during that time in her life.

It was the weekend, and one of my friends in the complex named Monique was going to a baby shower with her mom. Monique called and asked if I wanted to come along with them. Monique was the same age as me, heavyset with a dark complexion. No matter what time of the day, she was always sucking her thumb. We arrived at the baby shower around 4pm. The couple having the baby were in their mid-twenties. They were having a baby boy. The place resembled a banquet hall and was decorated very nicely in blue and white. There was a lot of food, and people were arriving slowly but surely.

By night time, it seemed like a dancehall as opposed to a baby shower. The place was crowded. The good thing about that is she received a lot of gifts for the baby. Monique and I decided to get some food and sit close to the guys playing the music. I noticed one of the guys playing the music looking at me. I looked away, shy because I was actually attracted to him. I quietly let Monique know that the guy was looking at me and that I liked him. We continued to eat our food and giggle about it. About twenty minutes later, he came over to the table to talk with us.

After his first sentence, Monique's mom came over. She asked him if he liked one of us, which was very embarrassing. He said no, adding that he was only speaking to us. In her loud voice, she replied, "They are not allowed to talk to boys." She then looked at us and said, "I don't want you talking to any boys. We should focus on studying our books." Monique's mom was a tall, heavy set, dark, loud Jamaican woman. She spoke her mind anywhere, any place, any time.

Embarrassing us was not a big deal for her. Anyhow, the boy did go back to playing music. For the remainder of the night, I kept my eye on him and on Monique's mom. It obvious that the boy and I liked each other. Before the night ended, I was able to write my beeper number on a piece of paper and sneak it to him. He let me know his name was Devoid.

Devoid was older than Prudence by two years. Prudence looked like a boy compared to Devoid. About a week after the baby shower, Devoid came to meet me in the park near my house. He had on blue jeans and a grey button-up shirt. His shirt was a little more than halfway buttoned up, causing his chest to show. I thought to myself, *He is a man*. Prudence did not have hair on his chest, and Devoid did. Sadly, I was in heaven knowing that a man actually liked me. I was very shy when speaking with him. Devoid and I spoke consistently on the phone. Some days he would even pick me up from school.

Devoid had worked at a shipping company for about six years. He already had one child, and he was very experienced. After being with Devoid for about six months, I learned that he had another girlfriend and that she was three months pregnant. I wanted to leave, but I also thought I was pregnant. I was absolutely crushed. Two weeks later my period came, so I knew I was not pregnant. I was disappointed. Not because of love, but because I wanted a baby. Devoid did not know about my prior miscarriages. I kept them to myself. I decided one day after school to tell Devoid that we could no longer be together because he had another child on the way. He left work and came to my house.

He told me that he loved me and I would not be doing his baby mother a favour, because if he could not be with me, it would be with someone else. He made it clear that the someone else would not be her. I should have ran, but being young and inexperienced, he definitely convinced me. I decided to stay with Devoid. After about one year, Devoid got into trouble with his boss at work. His boss fired him. I was still in school, and shoplifting had become my new hustle. Devoid had a car, so he started to go with me on the road after school. Since he had a car, we were able to go many places and to make more money. After about a year and a half of pursuing my degree, I dropped out of school and decided to hustle with Devoid. Whatever money was made we would split in half between us. I began to feel like I had found the perfect boyfriend.

Chapter 14

I was nineteen years old. I would have completed a degree in social work if I stayed in school. I did complete my internship, and I only had four classes left to get my degree. Having a boyfriend, money, clothes, and having my first child meant so much more to me. Devoid and I had been living together for about six months. We decided to get an apartment together because it would be easier to go on the road to hustle, and we thought we were in love. I say "thought we were in love" because I can now say that living a dishonest life together can never be love. What we actually loved was the life we lived. I felt like a grown woman who had all the answers. Sadly, even though I had my first apartment, a new boyfriend, nice clothing, and money, my depression worsened. I can now say that I let my miscarriages control my life.

I was with Devoid but not in love with him. I was too concerned about having my first child than truly getting to know him. Our day consisted of waking up around 12pm, going on the road, coming back home at around 11pm or 12am everyday. We partied a lot on the weekends and hung out with friends until very late. One year after being with Devoid, I decided to start having unprotected sex with him regularly. I didn't stress about getting pregnant, though I learned that when you don't try to get pregnant is when it happens fastest. About five weeks went by, and I decided to take a pregnancy test. Sure enough, I was pregnant. This time, I went to my fourth hospital and let them know about my prior miscarriages.

The doctors said I was considered high risk and that I would have to take baby aspirin to thin my blood. This pregnancy I will never forget. I bled in the beginning like in my prior pregnancies. I gained strength as well from the thought of possibly miscarrying; it helped me to be happy but not to get my hopes up of having a baby. During this pregnancy, I was very happy and did not let the bleeding get to me. I bled up until twelve weeks. After that the bleeding stopped. I was in heaven during this pregnancy. I bonded with my baby. It was like the baby was already born.

When I lay on my back, I would rub my stomach and read to the baby, and the baby would kick. When it was time to sleep, I would tell the baby it was time to sleep, and the kicking stopped. Only the Lord knows the bond that I had with that baby. I was eighteen weeks pregnant. I woke up one morning and we had intercourse. I took a robe his mom had given me for Christmas and threw it over me to run to the bathroom. I came back into bed and wrote a poem about how happy I was to be having my first child. About one hour later I felt water running between my legs. I told Devoid I thought something was wrong because I was peeing on myself. Devoid helped me get ready and rushed me to the hospital up the block from his home. When I arrived at the hospital, they put me in a wheelchair and immediately brought me up to delivery.

The doctors did a sonogram. I saw my baby moving and the heartbeat. The doctor held her head down, then looked up at me. She said she would have to dilate me and take the baby, that my water had broken, it was too early, and the baby would not survive. My body immediately began to heat up. I felt like I was going to faint. I stared at the doctor, speechless. There was a moment of silence between us. She shook her head again, stared back at me, and said she was sorry. After about three minutes, I was able to speak. I asked her if there was anything she could do to prevent this. She said no, then added that it was weird that my water broke so early.

I told her we'd had intercourse prior to my water breaking, and she said that would not cause my water to break. I said, "Please don't take my baby."

The doctor said she was sorry and that once the water broke there was nothing they could do because it was too early. I lay there, helpless and frozen. Another doctor came in and said they would have to dilate me. I really didn't know what that meant at the time. The doctor then placed some little sticks that resembled tiny icicles in my vagina. The silent tears never stopped flowing. I was nervous, confused, and in disbelief.

After about one hour, I started to feel contractions. The pain came on about every ten minutes. I was more confused as to why I had to go through that pain. I screamed until the pain stopped.

The nurse said, "This is only eighteen weeks, and you can't handle it. How would you have handled the pain at nine months? It would have been worse."

The doctor put her two fingers in my vagina, adding to the pain. I was giving her a hard time because the pain was unbearable. She told me she had to take the baby out. I finally let her get in. I pushed out my dead baby. The doctor took the baby, then she came to take out the afterbirth. They started to clean me up. The hurtful reality finally hit me. I'd experienced natural birth, but to a dead baby.

I asked the doctor what the baby would have been. She said it was a girl. Today I can still feel her kicks. I still think about her, and I'm not sure why, but I have moments where I try to imagine what she would have looked like. I missed the bond we created. It was like she was born and alive already and living life with me. It felt like losing a loved one that you have been around for years. It felt like a part of me was missing.

Chapter 15

I lay in the hospital bed, frozen. I was there for two days. I went into a dark life. I had thoughts of suicide, anger, hatred towards myself, and worthlessness. I thought abnormal thoughts, and then I would go blank. I didn't have any appetite, and the kind of depression I encountered was a kind where I could walk in front of a car, get hit, and not feel any pain. When I got out of the hospital, I tried to put the best appearance out there to avoid confrontation with the people who knew I was pregnant. Of course, people would want to show their sympathy, but I figured if I appeared okay, it would not be for more that one minute. I just wanted to be left alone. It was obvious that I was messed up.

As the days went by, my dress code changed. The colours were completely off and never matched. I wore more clothing than I needed to. My face showed how I was feeling at all times. I was more quiet than normal and I didn't smile; indirectly, my head was always held down when walking. Devoid, I believe, was hurt by the loss as well, but handled it in his own way. We did not have a relationship that involved a lot of chemistry, so there was no support between us in that way. Based on his actions, he was hurt but tried to put out the best appearance as well. I think most men are horrible at accomplishing that. Their body language usually gives them away.

About one month after the miscarriage, Devoid came to me and said that he believed the baby was still at the hospital. He assumed the doctors tell you that you miscarry, but what they really do is take the baby. I thought about it, and even though I thought it was unreal, I hoped that he was right. He said all we had to do was go to the hospital and ask for baby Isaiah. Isaiah was my last name. The doctors always called the newborns by the mother's last name.

We decided to go back to the hospital, and we went up to labour and delivery and asked one of the doctors for baby Isaiah. She replied and said, "When was the baby born?" She looked in a book I believed that had all the newborns' names, and she then said there was no baby Isaiah. She asked when the baby was born, and I said about one month prior. She said the baby should be home. I said okay, and left the hospital.

We were both disappointed, but I guess it all came with the territory of losing a baby.

I went back into the stores, and my shoplifting got worst. I stole what I did not need, want, and whatever I could get away with. I even stole a microwave, pots, and vacuum cleaners. As long as I could lift it, I was leaving the store with it. I did not fear jail, security, police, or anyone. My thoughts at the time were that there were only three places I could end up: jail, my grave, or my home, and I was okay with either one. As the days went by, I gradually got the urge to try again. This time, I decided to tell Devoid that I wanted to try to have a baby. He was okay with that. We were making money and we had our own place, so I figured why not try?

My mom had no clue what I was going through, and I made sure not to tell her. I did not want her to worry or to tell me that I was young and that I had my whole life ahead of me. After two periods, I chose to start trying again. I convinced myself that if I could bring a baby to eighteen weeks, I could bring a baby to term. I was very fertile. After my fourth miscarriage, I got pregnant one month after my second period. I learned that once I felt like I was okay and my body could handle the pregnancy, it was okay to go along with it. During this pregnancy, the bleeding started at six weeks up until sixteen weeks. At twelve weeks the doctors decided to put a cerclage in, a stitch in the womb to keep it closed. Women who miscarry more than two times usually get the cerclage procedure done. They informed me that it would take one week for the cerclage to heal.

As the days went by, my thoughts of having my first child prevailed over my fears of reality. I continued to bleed, and I knew that I was possibly going to miscarry. During this pregnancy, I stayed home most of the time. I ate and watched movies. When I was tired of lying on my back, I would go online and research miscarriages or download music. The doctors informed me that I was not allowed to have intercourse at any time during my pregnancy. One day I was home alone, about thirteen weeks pregnant, and I decided to walk around the house to give my body some exercise. I figured I would be ok. After about ten minutes, I started to bleed. I bled enough to believe I was going to lose my baby. I panicked and returned to my bed. Whenever I was going to miscarry, the timeframe from the beginning of the bleeding until I was sure I was miscarrying was about four hours. If after four hours the bleeding had slowed down, I knew I was not miscarrying. Walking was my enemy at the time. Sometimes even a walk to the bathroom would cause me to start bleeding. I thought, *If my body is used to lying down all day, the change in me getting up will cause me to bleed because that's not what my body is used to*. I kept that in the back of my mind. Being twenty years old on bedrest was very hard.

The day was October 23, 2001. I will never forget this day. It was also my mom's birthday. She didn't know I was pregnant. I'm sure I could have told her, but the pain from me assuming I could not have kids kept me from telling anyone but Devoid that I was pregnant. It was around three o'clock in the evening. I went to use the bathroom and was done urinating, but the blood slowly but surely came flowing. I held my stomach with one hand and the towel railing with the other. I cried painful silent tears. I spoke to myself, saying, "God, please no; God, please no; God, please no." As time went by, the bleeding got heavier. I already knew. About thirty minutes later, I put on two overnight pads and called the ambulance. I phoned Devoid and told him I was miscarrying and to meet me at the hospital.

Feeling the blood flow and the thought of losing my fifth child caused me to freeze. As I sat and waited for the ambulance, I didn't even bother to change my pad. I let the blood flow through my pants. Once the ambulance arrived, I walked to the door and was in a total mess. The ambulance guy looked at me like he'd seen a ghost. He stated that they'd received a call about someone miscarrying. It was more than obvious it was me. I was rushed to the hospital. Once again I was in labour and delivery.

The doctors did a sonogram right away. This time the baby was alive, of course with blood clot surrounding it, but sadly I was contracting very lightly. The doctors gave me probably about ten shots of something that was supposed to help me stop contracting and deal with the pain. A nurse told me that they were trying to help me keep the baby. As time went by, the pain got worse. I believed the doctors were trying to help me keep my baby, so I tried to bear the pain. After about two hours, I completely lost it. I turned over in the position of a dog, placed my head facedown on the bed, and I began screaming. The doctors came in and tried to help me calm down.

I finally gave in and begged them to take the baby out of me. The pain was unbearable, and they were not able to give me any more shots for it. I tried to relax, and the pain got worse. I yanked my IV out of my hand and ran into the bathroom. The shower looked similar to a stand-up shower. I turned the pipe on and wet my hair, and my whole body screamed in pain. Blood was everywhere. A few doctors came in and spoke to me. They said that for them to take the baby out, I would have to work with them, and we would have to go into another room. By then, all I wanted was the baby out.

I screamed and cried and cooperated with the doctors. I went back on the bed and allowed them to clean me up, preparing me to take out the baby. I did everything possible to deal with the pain. Before we left to go to the other room, a doctor came in and he removed my cerclage. I would never wish this pain on my worst enemy. At the time I was very thin. I weighed about 124 pounds. Everything that was going on took a toll on my tiny body.

Chapter 16

When I arrived at the other room, Devoid was there. He hung around for about an hour, then he left. The pain got worse and worse. A doctor came in and wanted to go inside to take the baby. I would have to push. When he started, it was unbearable. I was totally against it. The doctors left me in the room for about twenty minutes. They were frustrated, and I understood why. I couldn't take the pain anymore. I decided to sit up. Because of how the bed was set, I was able to bend my legs onto something the doctor had left on my bed. I started to push, As the baby came out, I wanted to stop, but it was so painful I decided I had to keep pushing. Finally the baby came out, and the pain eased up tremendously.

I stared at my baby in disbelief. When the doctor returned to the room, my baby lay still between my legs on the bed. They removed the baby, and the doctor told me she had to take out the afterbirth. That was not painful at all. A nurse came in and asked me if I wanted to see the baby again. I said yes. I asked her what the baby would have been. She said it was a boy. I asked her to take a photo of him with my phone. I still walk with his photo in my purse today.

My mom and sisters surprisingly arrived. Devoid called my mom and told her. I had to play tough. Surrounded by my blood, my mom broke down. I tried to show her I was ok. I tried to get out the bed and use the bathroom. I passed out; I had lost too much blood. I had to have a blood transfusion. I stayed in the hospital for a few days. The day I left the hospital, my mom came to bring me home. Once again I tried to act like I was ok; I never wanted her to worry about me. I said to her, "Mom, it was a boy," and that I didn't want a boy anyway. My stomach and chest pained me, because deep inside I knew that was not true. All I wanted was a baby, and it didn't matter whether it was a girl or a boy.

Chapter 17

I stepped through the doors of the hospital. The breeze blew in my face. I felt empty, confused, and hurt. I had left the hospital five times empty-handed. We drove to the pharmacy to fill my medications. I usually sat and waited for them to be filled. It took about thirty to forty-five minutes. I spoke, smiled, and ate something—stewed chicken and rice that my mom had bought for me. I just wanted to go home to my apartment. My mom wanted me to stay at her home, but I was not willing to. I told her I wanted to go home and that I would call her. She dropped me at home, and I went and lay in my bed.

Devoid was out with friends, as usual. I took a shower and my medications. I didn't know how to feel. I thought, *Maybe my purpose on this earth is to shoplift*. It was the only thing I was good at.

I made a promise to myself. I promised to never begrudge anyone who was pregnant or who had a child, and to never let being unable to have kids cause me to hate, mistreat, or not help anyone, especially someone who was able to. Seeing other kids was hard. When it was a friend's baby shower, I gave the most gifts. I gave away a lot of gifts to kids for Christmas as well. Devoid had two kids. His first son then became my kid. I took care of him and loved him like I'd given birth to him. Many times I thought *What is the purpose living if I have nothing to live for?* That's when I wished to have a child of my own.

One day I sold some clothes to a businessman for his daughters. He owned a small tire shop. When I arrived with the clothing, we had a little chat. During our conversation, I learned that his shop was paid off, his house was paid off, he was married, and he had two beautiful girls. I thought this was a life I would love to have. I told the man that one day I would stop shoplifting because those store owners are people just like me, trying to be just like him. He look at me and smiled, then said, "You have a conscience. You're a good girl." That stuck in my head for the remainder of the day. I knew what the word conscience meant, but I decided to look it up anyway.

My thoughts after were that I wanted to do better, I wanted better, and I would have a baby. I actually told myself, "You're not a shoplifter, you're hurt because you cannot have kids." My moods fluctuated as days went by. Some days a song could change my mood from happy to sad and vice versa. Other things that had an influence on my mood changes were colours, especially when I encountered a room, store, office. Wall art also affected my mood. I still go through that these days.

It had been three months, and I decided to look for a special doctor where I could pay to have my child. With all the money I had saved from selling chocolate and clothes, I had a little more than $10,000 saved. I went home did my research, and found out the doctor I needed to see was a Reproductive Endocrinologist. I was curious to find out why I was miscarrying and if I would possibly be able to ever have children. I then went to the yellow pages. I look under Reproductive Endocrinologist, and there were so many numbers. I decided to close my eyes, and whichever name my finger landed on would be the doctor I would call. The name of the doctor my finger landed on was Dr. Hallelujah. I made sure to call the following day.

Chapter 18

Besides having my first child, I also stressed about owning my own business. I'd always had a vivid imagination. Whatever I desired in life, I imagined myself actually having those things or living that life. I would get the drive to go out and do whatever it took to accomplish my goals. Owning my own business was important, but not as important as having my first child. I wanted to open my own discount store one day, then I would expand and open a chain of stores. I knew my way of living was wrong, yet I wanted to be a store owner. I would not want people to steal from me.

I just couldn't find any other way at the time to feel happy. Dancing and music helped sometimes. I liked to blast music and dance in front of the mirror for hours. By the time I was done dancing, I would probably play dress-up for a little while, and then the sad feelings would come into my chest and haunt me, forcing me to remember how worthless and abnormal I was. It hurt so bad that I stopped crying. I felt like crying was for weak people and a waste of time. Crying did not help anything in my life at the time. I isolated myself within.

I was not connected to anything or anyone, not even Devoid. I was a quiet person who didn't feel love, but I still managed to put out the best appearance in front of people everyday. Within myself, I felt anger and hate. Not towards anyone, but towards myself. Some days I wished I was not born, I wished God would take me. I thought about suicide a lot. I remember one day going for my regular GYN appointment. It was obvious to my gynaecologist that I was not happy. I knew her thoughts, because she always asked a million questions.

This day she had me fill out a booklet of questions, basically repeating themselves but written in different ways. After I finished the booklet, she asked me if I wanted to take an HIV test. I shrugged and told her ok. She then asked me if the test came out positive what I would do. I responded in a non-caring way that I would take my medication. I told her that if it came back positive, there was nothing I could do about it other than to take my medication. As we continued to speak, another annoying question came up about suicide.

She asked what my thoughts were on suicide. I said, "People who try to commit suicide and are not successful are not successful because they don't want to die." I added that if someone really wanted to die, it was easy. My two examples were to jump off a bridge or to purchase a few bottles of pills and take them all before going to bed. She asked me if I had any suicidal thoughts, and I said no. The questions went on and on until I became frustrated. The doctor tried to recommend that I come in for counselling. I refused everything. I decided that I would not go back to the doctor for a very long time.

The next day I was anxious. I picked up the phone and dialled. The person who answered was female. I introduced myself, then explained my situation to her. I told her that I'd had five miscarriages, and I wanted to understand why. I added that I would like to have one child. The person let me know that I would have to come in and speak with the doctor, and it would cost me $400. I agreed to the cost and made my appointment. I started to feel a little hope, and kept myself busy from becoming too anxious.

On my appointment day, I was extremely happy all over again. The clinic was very big and beautiful, clean and welcoming. Other women who had problems having a baby were there. Some even had huge tummies. The lady at the front desk was very pleasant. I approached the counter and she automatically said, "Hello, how may we help you?" I let her know that I had an appointment. She had me fill out some paperwork, and I paid her the $400 in cash. As I waited to see the doctor, I imagined what it would be like to become a mom.

I pondered what it felt like to be nine months pregnant. I wished I was pregnant, with a huge tummy just like some of the other women. After forty-five minutes my name was called. I was twenty-three years old, but I looked seventeen years old. I could tell by the look on the doctor's face. His facial expression said, "What is this young girl doing in my office trying to have a baby?" I introduced myself, then he asked me to explain my problem to him. After explaining everything, he was determined to help me. I felt great. He told me to go and get pregnant, and as soon as I conceived I should come back to see him immediately. As I left the doctor's office, I quietly said to myself, *Instead of saying why me, say why not me?*

Chapter 19

I went home and gave Devoid all the good news. I told him I'd found a doctor, and he was going to help me have a baby. Devoid was not really a family guy—he was not even the romantic, loving kind of boyfriend. He was materialistic and into his friends. Sometimes I thought he was around because of the fancy life we lived. I wouldn't let it bother me, because my main concern was having a baby. We were making money, and he had a penis. He also went with the flow. Within one month of my appointment, I became pregnant. This time I didn't try to get pregnant; I basically cleared my mind of getting pregnant. I thought positive thoughts daily in the assumption that I would become a mom soon.

My imagination of course influenced that, and I partied and had a lot of intercourse. I called Dr. Hallelujah's office and told him that I was pregnant. He told me to come in the next day. I arrived at his office at approximately 9am. He joked and told me that I was the most fertile woman he knew. I said, "Fertile, but infertile." He said, "We will do our best to help you achieve your goal." He put me on a blood thinner called Heparin. It was delivered with a needle I had to take—if I am remembering correctly—once a day.

This was supposed to help my blood thin in order for it to flow from me to the baby without clotting. This pregnancy ended in three weeks. I called Dr. Hallelujah and let him know I'd lost the baby. By then I was immune to losing my babies. He ran a few blood tests prior to my sixth miscarriage, but nothing came back negative. Anxious to have a baby, I waited for one menstrual cycle and then I started to have unprotected sex. I was convinced that Dr. Hallelujah was going to be able to help me.

Devoid and I had still been hustling through it all. We saved up a good amount of money and decided to take a trip to Barbados to visit his family. We went for one month. We partied and toured the place most days. It was my first time visiting Barbados. The country was beautiful, with a lot of beaches and great food. I met a lot of wonderful people and tried a lot of different foods. I loved the music, and his family was very welcoming. The trip to Barbados was well deserved and definitely what I needed after all I was going through. When I came back about two weeks later, I noticed that my period didn't come, and I took a pregnancy test. Sure enough, I was pregnant.

I called Dr. Hallelujah immediately. Just like the first time, he told me to come in the next day. I arrived at his clinic at around 9am. Dr. Hallelujah called me into his office, handed me a package, and told me he was referring me to another doctor who was willing to help. He said the cost to have my baby would be $2500. I did not have a job at the time, so I did not have insurance. I did have Medicaid. Dr. Hallelujah said they would let Medicaid pay for whatever Medicaid could pay for and I would have to pay for my medications and the $2500. The package had information about pregnancy, pamphlets, my cost, and my new doctor's name, phone number, and address. Dr. Hallelujah made an appointment for me two days later. He said the doctor would be expecting me.

Chapter 20

By this time my mom knew most of what I was going through, and she supported me 100%. My mom, Devoid, and I went to see the new doctor. His name was Dr. Best. We all sat in his office and spoke about my situation. He gave me a paper with a list of thirty-one different blood tests that I was to get done. He let me know that Medicaid would pay for it and that I was to go to a place where they did blood work as soon as possible. Once the blood work results came in, they would forward them to him. He told me that at my next visit I would have to have some money. He was willing to let me choose what amount that would be and how I wanted to pay off my balance. I asked to pay $500 for my next visit and $100 every week.

I would have to see Dr. Best once a week for a sonogram and for a progesterone in oil shot that he would give me. He also let me know that I could not start the progesterone in oil shots until I was twelve weeks pregnant. He stated that he would have to place a cerclage in my uterus. Dr. Best did a sonogram. He said I was six weeks pregnant. He showed me that there were blood clots surrounding my baby. Things started to make sense. After signing all the paperwork, my next appointment would be six weeks away.

For the next six weeks I bled on and off. I prayed from time to time, and I took things lightly. I knew that I had to make it to twelve weeks for Dr. Best to help me. I bled daily, but I was hopeful. Even though most of my days were painful, hope always found its way to me. That's when my drive for greatness kicked in. I spent most of my days watching TV, eating healthy, and taking my iron pills and folic acid. My mom was so supportive; she called every day to make sure I was ok. I made sure to stay off my feet as much as possible. I was extremely sick and spitting so much I had to walk around with a bucket everywhere I went. At about ten weeks pregnant, the bleeding had gotten heavy.

Devoid was at work one day, and I believed I was miscarrying. I got up and put a plastic bedcover underneath me. I called my mom and told her that I was bleeding and to please hurry over. Devoid did not know that I had given my mom an extra set of keys for our apartment. My mom arrived at the apartment about thirty minutes later. She lived about ten minutes away. When she came into the room, she saw me lying in my own blood. My mom looked like she was going to pass out. As for me, I felt like I was disappearing. She called the ambulance immediately and started to clean me up.

The ambulance came, and the bleeding continued. I had to play tough, because that was my way of letting my mom know I was ok. I didn't like to see her worry. I stayed calm and cooperated with the ambulance guys. I was rushed to the hospital, and they took me in right way. After explaining my situation to the doctor, she decided not to do the sonogram vaginally. The bleeding had slowed down by this time. Shockingly, I was not miscarrying. She did the ultrasound on my stomach. She showed me the baby's heartbeat and said my womb was still closed. Besides the bleeding, everything was ok. I was sent home. My mom wanted me to stay with her, but I refused. I knew it would be easier to be sad if I was home. I did not want her to worry about me. I went home and took a shower. The bleeding continued, but it was not so heavy.

Chapter 21

I was eleven weeks pregnant. One week away from seeing Dr. Best again. The bleeding started to pick up. This is when I learned what FAITH was. I could have panicked, as usual. Instead, I went down on my knees and my head fell low. Tears ran down my face. All the tears I held in came running down. The disquieting emotions came out. I closed my eyes and began to pray, interrupted by thoughts of losing my baby. I cried out to the Lord and asked him, "Please, Lord, don't let me lose my baby." I begged the Lord to let this one, just this one, please come. I was not finished. I said, "Lord, if you bless me with this child, I promise to stop shoplifting. I will get a job and be a better person. I will be the best mom to this child."

I continued to cry. When I was all cried out, I felt a sense of comfort within. I had no clue why. I was confident. For my days going forward, I was able to worry less. The bleeding had a mind of its own. Some days it was heavy, some days it was light. No matter what it was, it was put in the hands of the Lord. I just didn't feel the need to worry anymore. I was tired of hurt and disappointment. I decided to convince myself that all I was going through was normal.

It was twelve weeks, and I was anxious, excited, and determined to get to Dr. Best's clinic. My mom, Devoid, and I arrived at 8am. I signed my name and took a seat. The girl at the counter called me and told me I had a payment to be made. I gave her $500 cash.

She then told me it would be $100 every week going forward until I paid off the whole $2500. I agreed, and Dr. Best then called me in. He did a sonogram and showed me where two huge blood clots surrounded my baby as well as small ones. He let me know that out of all my blood work, one test came back positive. It was positive for Antiphospholipid Antibody Syndrome. Antiphospholipid Syndrome is an autoimmune disorder where your immune system produces antibodies that mistakenly attack your own tissues and organs. When I got pregnant, my immune system recognized my baby as a foreign invader and in return attacked my baby, causing me to miscarry.

Dr. Best gave me my first shot of progesterone in oil. He told me I had to make an appointment for the following week. He also gave me a prescription for the progesterone in oil and needles, which I would bring for every visit. It was a very tiny needle, with which he applied a shot to either side of my butt cheeks. After leaving Dr. Best's office, I went home. Devoid and my relationship was just ok. He was not staying home with me, and that's what I wanted and needed. I decided to go and stay with my mom. My mother was extremely happy with my decision. I was happy with my decision as well. Mommy treated me like a queen. I got breakfast, lunch, dinner, tender loving care, and the support I needed, even when I rebelled and didn't do something she wanted me to do.

Two days after getting my first progesterone in oil shot, I was lying in bed. My mom had just finished giving me lunch. I fell asleep for about one hour. I woke up and went to the bathroom. I urinated, then started to pass huge blood clots. I panicked for a second, then decided to stop. I started to count. I passed about twenty-five blood clots. I whipped up, put on a pad, and decided to go back to sleep. I knew the incubation period for a miscarriage was about one hour. If the bleeding slowed down after one hour, it was most likely a false alarm. I went back to sleep, and when I woke up, the bleeding had stopped completely. I then knew that I was not miscarrying. As the days went by, the bleeding completely stopped, or was no more than what you would call spotting.

Chapter 22

It was the fourteenth week of my pregnancy, and it was my second appointment with Dr. Best. I was prepared. I had my progesterone in oil, my needle, and my $100. Just like the last visit, I signed in, paid my fee, and waited with my mom. Dr. Best called me in and did a sonogram. He asked how I was feeling. I told him the bleeding had slowed down a lot and that I'd passed about twenty-five blood clots while using the bathroom. He smiled and showed me the sonogram. By the grace of God, the blood clots surrounding my baby were all gone. He pointed to the screen and showed me where some of the blood clots had been. They were no longer there.

Tears came to my eyes. They were tears of joy. Once again, faith had made me stronger. Dr. Best then said he would set up an appointment for my cerclage to be put in. I would go to the hospital that he was affiliated with to have it done. Women are born with estrogen and progesterone. Progesterone is what gives a woman her womanly characteristics and plays a big role in her carrying a baby to term. I was not born with the right amount of progesterone to accomplish this.

Soon after, I woke up to a phone call. Dr. Best called to let me know that he had scheduled an appointment for my cerclage, and it would be one week from the day of the phone call. I was very happy, but as the days went by, I experienced so many emotions.

Some days I was extremely happy and anxious, and some days when it hit me that I was still pregnant, I felt like it was too good to be true, and I would then become sad. Most days I panicked and checked my underwear to monitor my spotting. I focused on seven months. I told myself that I would try to pray and relax until seven months. The reason I chose seven months was because I knew that most premature babies born at seven months had a better chance at surviving.

I also decided not to think about my pregnancy, but to just be pregnant and pretend that I was normal.

I was fifteen weeks pregnant, and the next day I would be getting my cerclage emplaced. I had to be at the hospital for 8am. When I arrived at the hospital, I was told to go to the fourth floor. When I got out of the elevator, I arrived at the ICU. I went to the desk and gave the lady my appointment slip. She told me to have a seat. About one hour later, I was called into a room. The doctor explained to me all that was going to happen and showed me how the room was prepared and ready for my procedure to be done. I undressed and lay on the bed.

They let me know that I had to have a GYN done before the procedure and then I would be put to sleep. A few hours after my procedure, I woke up and was very nervous. The thought of them going inside my vagina made me uncomfortable. I knew the slightest thing could cause me to start bleeding. I felt a slight pain in my vagina and my stomach. I relaxed and prayed. I would have to urinate before I left the hospital. The instructions I was given were: no intercourse, and bedrest for one week, which made no difference because I had been resting for nine months and kept my feet up as much as possible. These instructions were to help my uterus heal properly. Going forward, I continued to keep my

HIDINGappointments every week and follow Dr. Best's orders until about eighteen weeks pregnant.

Chapter 23

There were no blood clots surrounding the baby after passing the twenty-five blood clots. They never returned. The bleeding was the most stressful thing. The bleeding continued on and off. After paying attention to my body and the bleeding, I decided that 100% bedrest was not a good thing. I would say 70%, but not 100%. By this time I'd become frustrated and sad. I followed all Dr. Best's orders, but lying in bed all day every day was hard. I was bored, and I thought way too much about everything. My negative thoughts outnumbered my positive thoughts.

The most stressful part I noticed was if I got up to use the bathroom, I started to bleed. If I got up to shower, I would start to bleed. If I got up for food, I would start to bleed. Sometimes if I even sat up, I would start to bleed. The bleeding would always cause me to panic. For the next few hours, I'd worry I was going to miscarry. I went through that up until I was eighteen weeks pregnant. That was mental and physical torture for me. I lay on my couch one day staring at the ceiling. I said to myself, *The reason I keep bleeding when I try to do light things is that my body is not used to it. What my body is used to is me lying on my back or side all day.*

I decided I would listen to my body. For example, if I had to urinate, no matter how bad I had to go, I would stay put, relax, and wait until I felt like my body was ready for me to get up and walk to the bathroom. I practiced this with everything I did. Even if it was to pick up a piece of paper. I relaxed and waited until my body felt ready to get up and pick up that piece of paper. Practicing this caused my bleeding to slow down tremendously, and eventually it stopped. I was in heaven, and I felt normal. I tried to pretend that I did not have all these complications.

I had finally encountered twenty weeks of being pregnant. Things for me were ok. Dr. Best told me he would reveal the sex of the baby the next day, and I was excited. I turned to my mom for support, and she was always there. My mom and I arrived at Dr. Best's office. We were both excited. He called me in and told me to lie on the bed. I closed my eyes and prayed, asking the Lord to bless me with a baby girl. If I was blessed with a boy, I would love him just the same, but I wanted a baby girl badly. Dr. Best measured the baby's arm, legs, head, etc. He also placed a long needle in my belly button to make sure the baby did not have any deformities. Finally, he showed me between the baby's legs and let me know that I was having a baby girl.

The feeling I had within was unexplainable. I wanted to jump up and scream, but instead I covered my mouth. Not only was I five months pregnant, but I was being blessed with a baby girl. Still trying to relax until seven months, I prayed and took things easy. Dr. Best gave me sonogram photos from when I was six weeks pregnant. I purchased a small album to store them. I had sonogram photos from six weeks to thirty-nine weeks. The photo he gave me at twenty weeks meant so much to me, because that's when I learned I was being blessed with a baby girl. The Lord continued to answer my prayers. I even had a photo of my baby with her eyes open while in my tummy.

One day I was home relaxing, my heart filled with joy. I cried happy tears and said, "Lord, this is my baby. No matter what, I will be the best mother to her, no matter what obstacles I have to face in life. I will be thankful, grateful, and love her with all my heart. I will get off the road and be a better person." Any person who feared the Lord would understand how serious this was. After leaving the clinic, I could not wait to call some of my friends. Devoid let them know that I was having a girl. My mom experienced it all with me, and she was happy as well. Besides my daughter, the Lord had blessed me with the best mother in the world.

It was Saturday morning, and I decided that I wanted to continue to work with my body and get used to doing things. I should still have been on bedrest, but I had been doing well with my new remedy. I got ready and asked Devoid to take me to the mall. I wanted to get out and browse all the different baby clothing. It felt so good looking at all the baby products and the variety of clothing. I couldn't wait to become a mom. We walked around the mall for about forty minutes. While in one of the stores, I felt the bleeding start. I rushed to the register to try to pay for my items, but the bleeding got heavy. I told Devoid that I had to leave the store and go to the restroom. Devoid stayed behind to finish our transaction. By the time I arrived at the restroom, I'd soaked my pad. My body overheated, and I had to remove all of my clothing in order to cool off.

I lined the toilet with tissue paper and sat down for about ten minutes. I felt weak, light-headed, and hot. I always walked with pads, urinating and then changing my pads. I had to get back to the car where I could lie down with my feet up. I put my clothing back on, washed my hands, and left the restroom. I felt awful, and while walking through the mall I felt worse. The bleeding continued, and

I started to sweat more. I thought I was going to pass out. A lady approached me and asked if I was ok. My condition was obvious.

I let her know I was okay and continued on my way. I phoned Devoid and told him to meet me at the car. Going down the escalator to finally leave the mall, I was convinced that I was going to pass out, and that at least if it happened in the mall, someone would call for help and I would be rushed to a hospital. I was bleeding heavily and feeling weak and lightheaded. I made it to the car and lay down with my feet up. I didn't panic, although I was bleeding. I fell asleep until we returned home.

Chapter 24

It was mind over matter. I had to get my body used to taking long walks and doing light work. After my episode in the mall, the bleeding completely stopped. I continued to work with my body. By the time I was at seven months, I was cleaning, doing laundry, cooking... I even attended block parties with a chair that I travel with and baby showers. I was able to feel more normal and enjoy the rest of my pregnancy. My best friend at the time was pregnant as well. We were able to do things together. Through the storm, I definitely experienced some sunshine. Dr. Best had no clue that I was working with my body. Things were going well with the baby and with myself.

I was about eight months pregnant, and I was feeling light cramping. I went to see Dr. Best, and he told me that I was dilating. He told me to drink a cold beer. I was not into drinking, but I did drink half a beer. Sure enough, the cramping stopped. The following week, the dilating stopped and everything was fine. As time went by, I got impatient. I pondered what the baby would look like, and on becoming a mommy. I was anxious, excited, and nervous. With all the vomiting and not wanting to eat, I was not able to put on any pounds. Mommy changed that once I decided to stay with her. Before I conceived, I was 124 pounds; by the time my daughter was born, I was 134 pounds. Not much of a difference.

By the time I was at eight months, I was open to exposing my pregnancy to everyone . Because of shame, a possible miscarriage, and all that I had been through, I chose to keep my pregnancy as sacred as possible. I had a baby shower, which I honestly did not enjoy. I did have faith, and I did trust God, but I was still bruised from my past miscarriages. Sitting in my baby shower chair, I thought, *I'm celebrating having a baby with all these people and I'm not sure if she is going to be born alive.* All the gifts and the clothing—especially opening the gifts—made me sick to my stomach.

I couldn't wait for the celebration to end. I should have been happy, but I was not. I was scared. I was scared of losing my baby and of finally having my first child. I tried to keep calm and get involved anyway. If all the people celebrating with me only knew what I had gone through prior to the baby shower and how I was feeling, I didn't think they would be celebrating with me.

I had been so used to being sad that I didn't know how to be happy. I had every reason to smile, yet I pondered the past.

Chapter 25

Today marked thirty-eight weeks for my pregnancy, and also the day for my cerclage to be removed. Going forward, I would prepare myself for a C-section. Dr. Best and I decided it would be safest for the baby and me. I was one week away from giving birth and meeting my firstborn. I was excited and ready. I had to get a bag with a robe, underwear, comb, brush, lotion, a change of clothing for the baby to wear home, and a car seat. I had to stay in the hospital for four days after my baby was born. For the whole week I had been preparing, praying, and experiencing different emotions. It was finally going to happened.

I was finally going to be a mommy. I remember being told by a nurse at one of the hospitals that women who had Antiphospholipid Syndrome were not able to bring a child to term, and I was nine months pregnant. I was told that because of the repeated miscarriages, they would never give birth. With help from the Lord, I did not give up or give into that at all. I was stronger. That day, my life would change forever.

It was approximately 6 am. I was on my way to the hospital with my mom and Devoid. It was the day my baby would be born. I arrived at the hospital and was told to go to labour and delivery. I got in the elevator and pressed level seven. For some reason, my excitement turned to fear. I worried about what kind of pain I would have to bear. I had lost babies where I'd passed out because it was a very early miscarriage. I had experienced contractions, which were extremely painful. I'd even experienced vaginal delivery, but to a dead baby. Now I was to experience a C-section. I was told that I was going to get a bikini cut. With a bikini cut, my pubic hair would grow and cover it, and I would still be able to wear a bikini without my scar showing.

I was nervous and felt like breaking down. I arrived at a front desk and introduced myself. I was then told to go into a room. Dr. Best came in and greeted me. I had to sign two pieces of paper. He then looked at me, and in front of my mom and Devoid, he said, "You are a strong girl. You're like my daughter." I held my head down and said thank you. It felt great hearing Dr. Best say that. Thirty minutes later, Dr. Best returned to my room and gave me a robe to change into. He let us know that only one person was allowed in the room with me during the procedure. I chose my mom. Devoid left the hospital about ten minutes later. The feeling of wanting to break down came back. I was scared and nervous. It was almost unreal, what was happening. I glanced at my mom, and there was no way I was going to break down and show any kind of weakness to scare her. Instead, I spoke about the baby with her and waited patiently.

Chapter 26

Dr. Best came into the room to let us know that it was time. Two nurses also came into my room and covered me up. They rolled my bed into the surgery room. I was transported from one bed to another. I was told to sit up. Dr. Best told me that he had to place a needle in my lower back and that it was important that I did not move. The other doctors held me in position, and Dr. Best went in. That was painful for me, but over pretty fast. They turned me around, causing me to lie on my back. I was not able to feel my legs. I was completely numb. I was not able to see the kind of tools Dr. Best was using, but I knew he was cutting into my abdomen. Soon, with the help of the other doctors, they took my baby out of my stomach.

My baby was six pounds, eight ounces and healthy. I still remember and can hear her first cry. I can still feel my first silent tear flow down my face, as if it was today. A female doctor showed me my baby. I was in shock. I had a baby, and she was alive. The Lord had blessed me and answered my prayers. While in the hospital, I still panicked for the first two days. I didn't want to do anything wrong. I must have called the doctor about ten times within the first two days. If the baby made a sound that sounded weird to me, I would call the nurse. I got over that fear before leaving the hospital. On

December 7th, 2004, I finally left the hospital with my firstborn, my blessing from God, my beautiful baby girl Makayla Best.

Only the Lord knows what I had truly been through, the pain and hurt that I felt, the confusion, the embarrassment, the dark nights, (this list can go on). I can honestly say, it was all worth it. I prevailed. When I walked through the hospital doors with my baby beside me, I was a strong and spiritual woman who could accomplish anything through Jesus Christ. My faith was like a fortress, and that was a token that could not be taken from me.

PART 2
— What Is Life Like Now?

One whole week had gone by. Makayla had been staying with my mother. I loved my daughter dearly, but the responsibility that came with caring for a child started to kick in. I was young and she was my first child. I didn't know how to adjust. I figured I would let Makayla live with my mom, and I would have the freedom to do whatever I wanted. I would visit my daughter once a day. I was still going through the healing process, so I wasn't doing too much. I lay in bed and thought about hanging out with friends, partying, and maybe opening my business so I could put Makayla into a private school, open an bank account for her, and buy her all the wonderful things in the world. Then my house phone raing. It was my mom.

Mom: "Hello, Hannah. How are you feeling?"

Me: "I'm feeling much better."

Mom: WWhen are you coming for Makayla?"

Me: "What do you mean?"

Mom: "I gave you one week, and now it's time for you to come for your child. She will live with you, and you will take care of her."

Me: "But I thought she would live with you?"

Mom (screaming): "Come and get your child right now. I better not have to call you back."

Me: "Ok, I will be there soon."

I was crushed and angry. My mom did not live far from my home. I owned an Acura Integra at the time, which I'd purchased online for $1500.

I didn't want to have a baby without a car to get around. I made sure to purchase the car before Makayla was born. On the way to my mom's house, I had so many thoughts. I questioned myself as to why my mom would do something like this to me. I'd experienced losing a baby in the most horrible ways. I'd experienced pushing out my dead baby, inducing labour, and having a C-section with

Makayla. The last thing I wanted to experience was my baby being born and then possibly passing.

Tears rolled down my face. I thought about her dying from SIDS. We lived in an apartment building, and sometimes the heat came on for about fifteen minutes during the day and that was it. I feared her dying from the cold apartment, I feared her dying from me giving her the wrong amount of milk, etc. I thought I would never speak to my mom again. I felt like my mom was the best person in the world to care for her. I didn't want to make any mistakes. Thirty minutes had gone by, and I arrived at my mom's home. I wiped my tears and got myself together. When I got inside the house, Makayla was fast asleep on the bed. I decided to get her dressed and ready to leave. My mom assisted me in doing this. Mommy was smiling and jolly, but I was angry and confused as to why she couldn't just keep her. Before leaving, she gave Makayla a million kisses, making me more upset. She then said to me, "Yeah, she is your baby. You take her home and bond with her." I did not respond. I left and went home with my baby.

When we arrived home, it was around 9pm. I lay her on the bed and decided to sterilize all her bottles. Devoid came home about thirty minutes after we did. I let him know that my mom had told me to come for Makayla. He said ok. During the night, I did not get much sleep. I was more frustrated. The next morning, after giving Makayla her bottle, reality hit me. I opened her wardrobe, The amount of clothes that I had shoplifted was ludicrous. She wouldn't even be able to wear half of them. I also realized that raising a baby was more than dressing her up in pretty clothing. I decided to close my eyes and pray. I thanked the Lord for blessing me with my first baby girl, then I asked the Lord to help me not make any mistakes while taking care of her and to help me to not be afraid.

Chapter 28

The following day, I decided to organize things in a way that would make things easier for me and Makayla. We both lay in bed, and I made sure her Pampers and wipes were at arm's length, her bottles were sterilized, water was boiled and cooling in time for her first bottle for the morning, and that she was dressed warmly and cuddled in her thick pink fleece blanket. Devoid always left the house around 6am for work, and it would just be Makayla and I home. As I lay in bed, my mind ran. I thought that I wanted to heal quickly and would do whatever it took. I pondered being a normal mom. One who had to drop her baby at daycare and had a legal job to attend or her own business. I wanted to be that mom. I thought about opening my own daycare center. I decided to phone Devoid.

Me: Hey, are you busy?

Devoid: "Not really. What's up?"

Me: "I was thinking... with the money that we've both saved, how about opening a daycare center? We can pay for our parents to take the classes, including me, and we have a newborn. It would be perfect. You have a job, and with the daycare, we would also have our own business."

Devoid: "We cannot afford a daycare."

Me: "We've lived together for five years, and we were able to afford everything else. Why can we not afford a daycare? We can combine our savings and make it happen."

Devoid: "NO, we cannot afford a daycare. I am going to buy a tractor trailer."

Me: "But I cannot drive a tractor trailer, and that's not what the plan was."

I was three months pregnant with Makayla, Devoid and I decided to go on the road extra early. We drove to another state. The rent was due, and the car payment and all the bills were piling up. We went from mall to mall. It was the last mall where we got caught for shoplifting and were arrested. My bail was $3,500, and Devoid's bail was $5,000. Thank God for my younger sister; we only spent the night in jail. She contacted a bail bondsman, and we were released the next day. The case stretched out for about one year. By the time we encountered the deadline for a decision about what was going to happen to us, Devoid was in the process of getting a job with the shipping company.

The day of the court date, the lawyer and Devoid pulled me aside. In order for Devoid to get his job, he could not have any recent priors. Also, to get his citizenship would be a problem. They both suggested that the case get dismissed against Devoid, and I took the case because I was a citizen. Devoid also said, "It's all good," because he would turn around and help me. After five years living together, hustling together and having a baby, I figured, why not help him?

Chapter 29

Months had gone by, Devoid had transitioned to another person. He was working at his new job, he'd leased a brand new BMW jeep, and he'd taken out a loan to finance his tractor trailer. He did not include me in anything. I started to feel like an outcast. I said to myself, *No matter what, I will help him get his tractor trailer on the road.* He worked from 8am to 8pm, so he did not have the time to do these things. After all I'd gone through, he never once made me feel appreciated for having his first baby girl or for all that I had done for him. I stood by him anyway.

One morning I was not sleeping, but I was still lying in bed with my eyes closed. Devoid woke up to a phone call, and based on how the conversation began, I could tell it was one of his friends. His friend was letting him know that he was considering marrying his girlfriend. It was obvious that the friend went on to ask him when was he going to get married. I remember it clearly as if it was today. Devoid responded that the ring didn't fit. I was in shock. I decided to continue to pretend to sleep.

I waited for a week to go by. I then went to Devoid and told him that I had a question to ask him. I told him it was about one of my close friends named Keisha. I said Keisha overheard her boyfriend speaking on the phone with his friend about marriage. His friend asked him when he was going to marry her, and his response was,

"The ring don't fit." I went on to ask Devoid what men mean by that. He clearly stated that it meant she was not the one for him. I flipped it and let him know that it was not my friend but him who I heard say it to his friend a week ago on the phone. Devoid's face looked like he'd just seen a ghost. Then his egoistic and prideful self kicked in. He denied saying it, and after ten minutes of going back and forth, he let me know that he would put me out but knew I had nowhere to go.

I told him he must have forgotten where he was coming from, because I was the one who'd found the apartment when he was living with his mom, and we'd both furnished it and been paying all the bills. What happened was Devoid was high on his horse and self-centered. He felt that because we used his name to get the apartment as far as paperwork was concerned, all of a sudden he owned the apartment. They say vanity can change people, and as this relationship continued I totally experienced it, from the disrespect, the coming home late at nights, the many different women, the fights, the evil mother-in-law... the list goes on.

I still managed to hold on, waiting for the change that most women wait on, when most of the time it turned out that you were only waiting on a disappointment. Most people would ask why you went so hard and waited. I did it because of my daughter, and I also felt that he would be the best person the build the rest of my life with. I took a case for him. I wanted him to help me just like I helped him. As time grew, I grew more unhappy. I did what I had to do to take care of Makayla. When my hurt became intense, I did what I did best: I spoke to myself for hours.

When I was around five months pregnant, Devoid and my apartment was robbed. I feared being home alone. Devoid hung out late nights and sometimes until broad daylight. I would talk to myself in order to not fall asleep, and I found comfort in doing that. If I did dose off and a pin dropped, it would awaken me. Some nights I would cry from being exhausted and afraid to sleep. I feared someone breaking in again and hurting me and my baby. Devoid did not know about this.

Chapter 30

One year had passed since Makayla was born. She was walking and doing so much. I had grown so much. The fear that I had when caring for my daughter had turned everything wonderful. I'm thankful that my mom did what she did by calling me to come for Makayla. It all makes so much sense.

After a C-section and a newborn one year later, I was 126 pounds and my stomach was as flat as a ironing board. My hair had grown past my shoulder and I was stunning for a mommy. Things between Devoid and I had become worse. It was like I didn't even know this man.

It was an early Monday morning. I woke up and let Devoid know that something was wrong. I told him that I didn't feel well. He looked at me without saying a word, and then he went through the door. My throat was sore and white, and my bones were aching badly. I felt very stiff.

I called my mom and she called the ambulance. My mom arrived at my house within about twenty minutes. I was in so much pain that I could not get up to feed Makayla. I told my mom that Makayla needed a bottle. She fed her for me. When the ambulance arrived, I was lying stiff and weak in bed. When I arrived at the hospital, the doctor looked into my throat and gave me two pills to take. After she was finished with me, I'm not sure why, but she looked at me and said, "Stress could kill you, did you know that?" I said no.

The medication did ease the pain a lot. I was in the hospital for about one extra hour, until I was given my discharge papers.

I called my mom, and she and Makayla picked me up. She then dropped me home and told me that she would keep Makayla and I should get some rest. I thought about what the doctor had said. It did click in my head that I was stressed, but I did not want to die. Once I got into the house, it was still light outside, so I decided to shower and get some rest. I woke up around 7pm. I looked in the mirror at myself and I heard a voice speak to me. The voice said, "You do not have to deal with this, you choose to deal with this." Still looking at myself in the mirror, I responded and "You're right, I don't have to deal with this." Then I added, "Look at me; I'm beautiful and nothing is wrong with me. Why am I dealing with this?" I decided to phone Devoid.

I said I'd decided that I was leaving. He responded, "You might as well because it is not working." I said to him to just remember that when I left, I was never coming back. I called my mom and asked her if Makayla could live with her for a while until I got my life together. My mom didn't ask any questions, but said of course. I told her I would pack up Makayla's clothing and drop it off. I then closed my eyes and asked God to help me so I would never have to ask Devoid for anything ever again. I looked around the apartment and decided I was leaving everything. I packed up my clothing and put it in a closet. I had some really nice silk polo sheet sets, so I took a few of those and gave them to my mom.

I had made a decision that I was not going to give up, and I was going to do whatever it took to give Makayla a great life. I was very hurt, because I'd made a promise to God that I would not go back on the road if he blessed me with a baby. At the time I couldn't find a job. I drove to many retail stores trying to find work, and nothing came through for me. I decided to go back on the road. I said to myself that God knew what I was going through and one day I would get it right and keep my promise.

Shoplifting became hard for me. I was scared of getting caught and feared doing time. Most of the time when I walked into a store it was like the president had arrived. The security guards knew me as well as the workers, they just couldn't catch me. I always followed the store policy. My money was running low and I was getting desperate. I had ended my relationship and could not raise my baby in jail. I was practically homeless.

Chapter 31

One week later, it was around 9pm when I pulled up to the gas station. There was a really good-looking guy who approached me and asked if he could buy my gas. With all that I was going through, I said ok. I asked him what he did for a living, and he told me he was into Freud. The first thought that came to my mind was to run. I didn't need to be affiliated with someone into a life i wanted out of. Then I remembered that I had no job, no money, and nowhere to live. I could have gone to my mom's apartment, but with six people (three adults and three kids) in a one-bedroom, there was no space for me to go back there. My daughter's father made life a living hell for me whenever I slept there. I decided to give in and date this new guy. He asked me what I was doing for the remainder of the night, saying that he and his friends were headed to the city for drinks and partying. I was not dressed up, but I looked appropriate enough. I was not into wearing dresses and heels anyway, and he was okay with what I had on, so we decided to park his car and drive my car to the city.

His name was Decent. He was tall and slim, with curly hair and a fair skin tone. He was from the West Indies, a beautiful country call Trinidad and Tobago. He had a very strong Trinidadian accent, but I understood him very well. Decent was a wonderful guy with a concept of life that was wrong. He was the man any woman would love to have as a husband. He was caring, loving, and honest, but extremely immature and dramatic. I thought good things about him, but after coming out of a hurtful relationship and all that I was going through, love was not on my mind. I was honest with him, and I let him know this. He was okay with that for a little while. We finally met up with Decent's friend at a twenty-four-hour parking lot. Decent's friends were loud, flashy, and cool. There were two cars and they paid for parking. Then we all got acquainted as we made our way to the club.

The party was more like a rave. It was in a building, they played techno music all night, and there were torches and people drinking and smoking. I thought to myself, *Am I in hell?* I was not into techno music, and I was not a drinker. Decent asked me what I would like to drink. I said I didn't know. I was not familiar with the different liquors they had. Anyway, Decent and his friends brought a huge bottle of what I can now say was Hennessey. He gave me a Hennessey with coke. It was absolutely disgusting, so I decided to take big gulps. I finished my drink in about five minutes. I was handed another one. I felt amazing. I felt all my worries go out the window. I danced and I laughed and I had a great time.

After the party, we went back to his home. Decent lived in a room at a friend's house. When we arrived, he started to play video games and I passed out. I think back periodically on my life and realize how the Lord has always been with me. I met an absolute stranger and went out and fell asleep in his bed without getting raped or even touched. When I woke up in the morning, I felt like crap. I had a hangover, and Decent was still sleeping. I was scared and sad. I missed my daughter, but I had to get it together. I just lay there, nervous. When Decent woke up, he asked me if I wanted to go home. I told him to walk with me to my car and that I would be right back.

I went by Devoid's and my apartment and took a shower. I still had the key to get in. I only went there when he was at work. When I arrived back at Decent's home, he told me that they were headed to the city to hustle. He asked me to come with him. Once I figured out exactly what they were doing, I decided to work with him. I hustled and saved all my money. One day Decent came to me and said we were going to a party and I was not allowed to wear jeans. By this time I was getting used to everyone and taking notes. We went to the mall, and Decent purchased me a nice dress with shoes and a bag to match.

My hair was always done, and I looked beautiful. I didn't know how to walk in heels, but I wanted to fit in, so I wore them anyway. I now was introduced to the life of upscale parties, restaurants, and drinking. We dressed up, drank, and partied most nights. I lied and told my mom that I had a new job and would visit once a week to see Makayla. When I arrived at my mom's, I made sure I had toys for Makayla and money for my mom for helping me with her. I tried to smile and make my mom assume I was the happiest girl in the world.

My new life of partying, shopping, and drinking was bittersweet. I enjoyed it, but at the same time it was a life I no longer desired to live, especially being involved in scams. No matter how much money I made or how much fun I had, the millions of toys I purchased for Makayla and everything it came with never made me feel satisfied or complete. I wanted to fall asleep with my baby girl every night and wake up to her every morning. I wanted to take care of her physically and stare at her all day. I decided to drink to ease the pain.

Chapter 32

It had been six months since Decent and I had been dating. Things on the streets were slowing down, scams were slowing down, and no money was really being made. One day I suggested to Decent that we should try to get legal jobs and find an apartment. Decent said he was going to hustle for the rest of his life. He did not have a Green Card, and he overstayed his time in America. I let him know that the last thing he wanted to do was to get arrested. Not only could you go to jail, but you could get deported. Decent was trying not to hear anything I had to say. Decent and I were on the road, and he let me know that we could move to another city named Vegas Island. He said his cousin owned a house out there and the cousin was never home. I agreed to make the move. After living there for about one month, it turned out the house was owned by one of Vegas Island's biggest drug dealers.

It was not the best place to live, but it was better than where we were staying before. We still lived in a room, but the house was much bigger, cleaner, and sacred. Living there, I witnessed prostitution for the first time. There was a pimp named Dollar, and he had a lot of women for sale. One of the prostitutes I spoke to called herself Clitexy. I asked Clitexy why she did it. She said she was trying to become a famous painter, and it was her only way of making money. Clitexy was from Russia, and she had a very strong accent. She said she did not have any family here. I wanted to ask her how she got here and whom she come to, but I did not bother. Clitexy had a few of her paintings there at the home, mostly naked women who looked sad or scared. I assumed they were images of how she felt within. The house was a one-family house with four rooms and a bathroom on the top floor, and the kitchen and dining room on the first floor. All rooms were always occupied.

One morning, I was using the restroom and playing with my cellphone when a call came in from Devoid.

Me: "Hello?"

Devoid: "Hi, how are you?"

Me: "It's your fault I'm going through this."

Devoid: "Where are you guys? I will come and get you both."

Me: "We will be okay."

Devoid: "You can come back home."

Me: "I will call you back."

I closed my eyes and began to pray. I asked God to stick with me and help me get through this storm so I would never have to go back to Devoid.

I would never be with or allow another man to treat me like he did. I then heard Decent calling me, yelling from the bathroom. I told him that I was coming, and when I arrived in the room, Decent said he needed to speak to me. He let me know that he would like for me to cook and clean for him. I almost fainted. I thought to myself, *This man is absolutely losing his mind.* By this time, I knew that Decent was not the man I wanted to be with and that I was not even into him in that way. I made it clear to him in a nice way, then asked him if I was his wife. He said yes. I said, "No, I am not your wife, and I'm surely not cooking and cleaning for you or anyone." I added that we were now living in a whorehouse, not a home where you could raise a family and be safe.

Decent started yelling and stated that he was paying $800 for us to live there and that I was ungrateful. I explained to him that I was not ungrateful, but why pay $800 a month for a room that was not yours? Decent thought that by moving into the drug dealer's home, he could make up for not wanting to quit hustling and getting a legal job. Decent even had the nerve to tell me that he would buy many toys so Makayla could come by sometimes and have them to play with. I then asked Decent, "When you buy all the toys for her to come here and play with, and the police possibly invade the home and find drugs, prostitutes, credit cards, and everything else illegal, what will you do with Makayla then?" I explained that they would not only throw me in jail, but they would take her from me. He replied, "The home is safe and has cameras," and that it was unlikely the police would ever show up there.

I began to understand that I was clearly speaking to a brick wall. Decent just did not get it. I would never feel safe with Makayla there. After going back and forth, I went downstairs and decided to cut hot dogs up and fry them with beans. Decent was more upset. I then said to him, "Now who is ungrateful?" I did like to cook, and I was good at cooking—mostly Caribbean food—but I was not in a position to play the wife role and live under those circumstances, I wanted a real family and a real life.

The next morning I woke up with so much on my mind. I wanted to live with my daughter so badly. I wanted to live a normal life. It was my birthday weekend and I was turning twenty-five-years old. I was not where I wanted to be, and I felt horrible. Decent and his friends decided that we were all going to go out that Friday night to celebrate. My birthday was not until the following Monday, but we decided to celebrate all weekend. I purchase a sexy fitted-lace dress from Marciano for $500 and a pair of Manolo Blahnik shoes for $700. My nails and toes were diamond studded, and I wore my hair straight. I felt like a princess. While on our way to the club, Decent said he had something for me to try. It was a white pill. At first I said no, then he said, "Come on, it's your birthday. Pop one with me." I wondered what it would feel like. I decided to do it.

Everyone was so excited. Another guy named Joe and I were the oldest out of the four of us. Decent was twenty-three-years old, and Joe's girlfriend Mariah was twenty-two. It made sense why everyone was so happy to take ecstasy pills. We all popped a pill with a beer. I sat there quietly until we arrived at the party. In my mind I felt like the pill did not work, because I didn't feel any different. When it was time to get out of the car and I stood up, I felt the effect of the pill. I thought I was floating, and I started to breathe hard. I must admit that it was an amazing feeling. Decent panicked, because I almost could not control myself. They gave me water to drink. I calmed down enough to get into the club. When I arrived in the club, they were playing techno music. I danced and climb on couches and was in a whole other world. We went at it all night. We had a lot to drink, and we partied until around 5:30am.

I woke up the morning, freezing cold. When I opened my eyes, I was lying in a hospital bed with doctors standing over me. The doctor asked me if I'd been drinking, even though It was obvious. I said no. The doctor then said, "Do you know that you could have been dead today and you would have not seen your twenty-fifth birthday?" I felt horrible, The doctor said, "Do you know that you were in a car accident?" I didn't even remember getting in the car, but I said yes.

My mom and sisters were outside, and the doctor called them in to see me. My mom had tears in her eyes. I told her that the other car hit us. I didn't even know what had happened. I asked them for Decent, and they told me that he had been arrested for drinking and driving. I went to stay with my mom for a few days until Decent got out of jail. Decent's cousin bailed him out, and he was out on the day of my birthday. Since my birthday was the day that Decent got out of jail, we decided to just stay home and relax.

I asked Decent what had happened. He said that we were all wasted, adding that he did consume a lot, but felt he was ok to drive. He said that by the time I got in the car, I was passed out. Joe and Mariah were smoking weed. He said he came to a four-way intersection, and a car ran the stop sign and hit him, totalling the car. He said my head hit the dashboard and I flew a back into my seat. Blood was gushing out of my head, and he had to use his shirt to put pressure on it. He phoned the police. Decent started to cry and say how sorry he was. He said I was lying there just crying. The ambulance got there pretty fast, and they rushed me to the hospital. They tested Decent's alcohol level and it was high, so they arrested him. The person in the other car ran off and left his car. We later learned that the other driver did not have insurance and was driving with a suspended license. I started therapy and ended up suing the other people and wining the case.

You would think that possibly losing your life would have stopped me from getting high, partying, and drinking, but it did not. I continued to party and drink, get high, and hustle in stores. Even though I was able to do whatever I wanted and get whatever I wanted, I realized something. It was about two months later when I woke up. We decided to prepare ourselves to go on the road. I noticed when I looked in the mirror how my face looked. I appeared very sleepy, even when I was not sleepy. I was breaking out, with huge bumps on my face. My hair looked thin, and my skin was very pale and dry. I did not look fresh and youthful anymore. By the grace of God, I wanted to make a change. I decided that I would stop taking ecstasy pills. I was not addicted to them, so quitting was not a problem for me, thank God. My drinking increased. It was like I drank more liquor to replace the ecstasy pills. Decent continued to drink and get high, and I decided that eventually I would get out of my unhealthy relationship with him.

Chapter 33

It had been about eights months, and Decent and I were still together, but not in any kind of loving relationship. I knew I wanted more out of life. I had been visiting my daughter, and as the months grew, my pain and hurt grew. I decided to sell my old Acura Integra and lease a brand new Jeep Infinity. I decided I wanted to pursue my dream of owning my own business. With the money I'd saved, I opened a discount store. I named my store Makayla's Discount Inc. The store was four-hundred square feet, which was very small for a discount store. As a first-time store owner, I did not know any better. I purchased products from different wholesalers to sell in my store. I basically sold health aids, beauty aids, electronics, hair products, detergent, party supplies, and home supplies. When purchasing these products, I learned that it was nothing like buying on the streets. The most you would make on your money was about 10%, and sometimes less. That was very disturbing for me. On the streets, you would purchase something for half price or bargain for less than half price. I expected the same thing when purchasing products legally from wholesalers. I was not discouraged, and I still pushed and decided to give it a try.

Makayla Discount Inc. was a small store, but I tried my best to make it work. I strongly felt that I'd made the right decision in starting my own business. I convinced myself that I would become very wealthy and then open a chain of discount stores. My awning resembled the colours of a candy cane. It was mostly white, with a variety of colours. It said Makayla Discount Inc., stated what I was selling, and included the address of the store and the telephone number. One month after opening the store, I realized that I'd made a huge mistake getting involved in a discount store and not educating myself about it.

My store was empty for the grand opening, which was very discouraging. I probably had five pieces of anything I advertised about selling. The look on the customers' faces when they entered the store was not encouraging at all. I had to turn to God. I decided to keep my faith, and I told myself that even if I didn't make a dollar for the day, I was going to be successful. I opened the store seven days a week, from 10am-10pm. I made about $100 a day. Some days I made $24 a day, maybe a little more, maybe a little less. I was exhausted by the long hours, so I decided to close on Sundays. Days turned into months. I was not making any money at the store. I decided to hire a friend of mine. Her name was Julie. Julie was a dark-skinned girl in her early twenties. She was heavyset, and a great friend who had been in my life for about seven years. I felt like I could trust her and that she was the perfect person for the job.

I went back into the stores, shoplifting things to sell in my store to make ends meet. Every morning I would open the store and wait for Julie to come in at around 10am. I would then leave. Most days were hard and depressing. I questioned myself as to how wrong it was to shoplift from another store to sell in my store, and to have to live that life in order to make ends meets. I held on to my faith and trusted God that one day I would get it right. Within a year of having my store, I tried a variety of things to avoid having to go on the road and hustle. I purchased plain t-shirts and designed them myself. I didn't have good equipment for this, so I used spray paint and regular paint to design them and sell them in my store. They didn't do too bad, but they didn't sell too well either. I then decided to write poetry, print it on a sheet of white paper, and place it in a picture frame to sell. No one was really interested. I then made mixed CDs to sell, and that did not work either. I was at the verge of giving up. I felt discouraged and uninterested.

It was a Friday night, and I decided to go to the liquor store and purchase a bottle of Grey Goose and a few bottles of Red Bull. During this time in my life, my moods were in control of my life. I could be happy and determined one minute, and another minute I was discouraged, doubted myself, and would just drink. That Friday night, I decided I was going to stay home and drink. I was overwhelmed with disappointment and felt hopeless, worthless, and like a failure. I repeatedly told myself this. That night I did not finish the bottle, but I did finish more than half the bottle. I drank and listened to sad music. Eventually I knocked out. I woke up the next morning and felt horrible. I had the worst hangover ever; I felt so sick that I couldn't eat anything. I had to go to the store. I dragged and dragged, but by then I honestly didn't even care. I got dressed to go to the store with the mindset of a person who has given up; I was finally ready to close the store.

Prior to going to my store, I was not sure what drove me to do this, but I stopped at another discount store to see how the store was set up. This discount store was very big, It had aisles, shelves, and even slotted walls. The store was fully stocked with products that were high-ticket items but being sold at extremely cheap prices. I said to myself, *How is that possible? How does this person even make money if he is able to sell these products so cheaply?* To make things more interesting, I learned that the store was black-owned. I was in awe. I decided to buy some of the things to sell in my store. I phoned my mom and told her to meet me at the store so she could witness what I'd learned and to help me with the bags.

I picked up about $100 worth of products. Still feeling horrible and discouraged, I walked over to the register. A man came over to the register to help me. My mom arrived during the transaction. I looked at the man and rolled my eyes. I assumed right away that he didn't trust me because of how many things I was purchasing. He asked me if I needed help bringing the bags to my car, and I replied no. He asked a second time and, already in a bad mood, I said no once again. Before leaving the store, I told my mom to ask the same man—whom I assumed was the store manager—where did they got their products from. After ringing up and bagging my things, the guy came out from behind the register. My mom approached him and let him know that her daughter had opened a store and would like to know who the supplier was for their store so she could purchase products from the same people. The guy let her know that he was the owner of the store and also a wholesaler. The products belonged to him. While my mother and the man conversed, I put the bags in the car. Once I was finished and returned to the store, my mom let me know that he was the owner. My thoughts went blank. I was shocked.

The man looked at me and asked me how old was I. I replied that I was twenty-eight years old. He then said, "You're twenty-eight-years old and you opened a discount store." I said yes. He was very impressed and immediately said, "I will help you." He invited me and my mother into the basement of his store. He said, "This is one of my small warehouses." He said I could take whatever I needed to sell and stock my store. I thought, *This man is crazy. He does not even know me.* I stood in the middle of the warehouse just looking around, staring at all the products. I didn't know what to do or where to start. I felt a little hope in my heart once again. I asked a million questions about how, what, where, and when. I learned that this man was making money and an honest living. I wanted the same thing. I was determined once again. I told myself I would become his friend and learn exactly how it was done.

He gave me a long cart to stock whatever I wanted. I took things in very small proportions. He then said, "I tell you to take whatever you want and this is what you take?" I didn't know what to say. He asked me for the address of my store, which was about ten blocks away. He said he would come and take a look at the store and bring some items as well. I agreed and left the store. I was encouraged and happy all over again.

The wholesaler's name was Phantom. Phantom was a tall, slim, fair-skinned, elderly man in his early forties. When Phantom spoke, he spoke with confidence, which was very intriguing to me. He was very prideful and hardworking. I later learned that he sold discount products to all the discount stores in the five boroughs: Brooklyn, Manhattan, the Bronx, Staten Island, and Long Island. About one hour later, Phantom arrived at my store. His exact words were, "You're going to need a lot of help." He let me know that my store was not only empty, but it was not set up correctly. He brought a few products to start me off: detergent, toothpaste, lotion, etc. He then let me know that he would stock the store for me. As I started to sell, I would pay him $500 a week. I felt like it was all unreal, but my dream was finally happening. As the days and months went by, Phantom and I gained a friendship. He stocked my store with everything and anything you could find in a discount store, from detergent, beauty aids, health aids, bathroom accessories, toys, electronics, nutrition bars, grills, pots... the list went on. There was not a huge walking space to shop, but I was happy the store was stocked with a variety of discounted products.

With all that said and done, I was still not making enough money to pay the bills, pay Julie, and pay him. After about one year, I decided to go on the road with Phantom and do wholesale distribution during the week, working at the store on weekends. I was spending less time at the store, and in some sense I left my friend to run it during the day. I would open the store in the morning and close the store at night. One night while I was on my way to the store, I received a phone call from Julie. Julie let me know that the store had been robbed. When I arrived at the store, the register was wide open and a chair had been thrown on the floor. Based on my observations, it looked fishy, but I thought that Julie was my friend. She let me know that some young boys had come in with a gun and stolen $80 out of the register.

I told Julie it was okay, and I closed the store. The next day, when I let Phantom know the details, his response was that Julie was stealing from me. I did not want to believe that, so I told him she was my friend. He said that he had been in the business for years, and he knew what he was talking about. Two weeks later, I arrived at the store a little earlier than usual. I don't stay long, and I let Julie know I would be right back. While walking to my car, my phone rang. It was my friend Rose. It so happens that I got caught up in the conversation and decided to sit in my car and talk to Rose.

From where my car was parked, I could see my store. While talking to Rose, I observed a guy in a black car pull up in front of the store. He went inside the store, and about fifteen minutes later he left with four bags, which he placed in his trunk. I told Rose I'd call her back, and I called Julie. I asked Julie how much money I'd made for the night. Julie said $4. I then asked Julie about four times if she is sure that was all the money I'd made for the night, and each time she said yes. I left my car and returned to the store. I asked Julie where the receipt was for the guy who had just left. Julie tried to tell me that there was no guy who had just come into the store. I let her know that I was outside the store sitting in my car. Julie was in shock, and she said she didn't have the receipt because she didn't charge him tax.

It was plain to me that Phantom was right and that Julie was stealing from me. I told Julie that she should not come back to work and we were no longer friends. After about two weeks, I hired a guy name Paul. Things didn't work out with Paul either. He was lazy and dishonest. After about one month, I let him go and decided to sell everything in the store to another man who wanted to open his own discount store. I did wholesale distribution full-time.

While doing wholesale with Phantom, I was able to gain my own accounts. There were so many stores that he could not get to, so I would sell to those stores. He was not allowed to sell to them, because those were my accounts, and that's how I made my money. Phantom basically taught me the wholesale business. I enjoyed doing wholesale, but I always felt like I wanted more independence. I was honest with Phantom during our time of working together; working with him was bittersweet. We did things by his time, his pace, and in his way. Sometimes I felt like I was stuck making an honest living and a decent income, but it was not my own business, not my dream. I wanted my independence back and to be able to do things my way. Because of an incident in my life in the past, I felt like I had to settle, and Phantom used that to his advantage.

I always assumed I would never be able to get a real job because of a fight I had in my past with a female who falsely accused me of stabbing her. We had an argument over a dance group I no longer wanted to be a part of, this became hostile, and we started to fight. Because of her losing the fight, she went inside the house, got a small knife, and stabbed me in the chest. I didn't realize it until my body started to heat up and my blood gushed out. I was rushed to the hospital and suffered from a collapsed lung. The doctors said that if it had been five minutes later, I wouldn't have made it. I was in the hospital for three weeks. While I was in the hospital, the female stabbed herself in the leg and told them that I'd done it. The case did turn around in my favour; however, I was charged with disorderly conduct. The judge knew I was innocent, but had to charge me with something to avoid me suing the police department for false arrest. My lawyer sued the detective who had arrested me. When I came out of the hospital, the detective told me to come down to the precinct to fill out paperwork. When I arrived, he handcuffed me to a chair for twenty-four hours. I was able to sue him for handcuffing me to a chair with open wounds, but we were not able to sue the police department.

Chapter 34

I was twenty-four years old at the time. My dream was to work with kids. During my time in college, I'd managed to finish my internship, and I had four classes left to complete my degree. I went to a group home and filled out an application. Based on the qualifications, I was fit for the job. It paid $10 an hour, was full-time, with benefits. I was in heaven until the day of the orientation. When they called you to come in for orientation, that basically meant you had the job. I was called, but I was not there for long.

I was called to an office and handed a letter stating that because of a prior arrest, I was not going to be able to get the job. I explained to the lady what exactly had happened when I was arrested. She explained to me that she believed me, then she told me something that implanted itself within me for the next few years of my life. She said, "If you know of someone who was arrested for assault, regardless of how the case went, if we hired them to watch your child, how would you feel?" She added that people were not concerned about how a case went, but they were concerned with what you were arrested for. Right then and there, I thought about reality. I said to myself, *She is right*. Regardless of the situation, I would not want someone like that taking care of my child. I told her I understood, and I left the office.

I told to myself that my life was screwed and I would never get a legal job. I had not assaulted anyone; I was the one assaulted and in the hospital for three weeks, and it was now affecting me getting a job. I was convinced that I had to own my own business in order to survive and take care of my daughter. I told myself that I would never apply for a job again and have to face that kind of embarrassment. Days went by, and I decided to go to the lawyer who helped me with my case. When I went to his office I saw him and explained what had happened, that my record stated I'd done jail time. He told me that the time I had been handcuffed to the chair was the time served. I was crushed. I couldn't believe what I was hearing. I left his office in tears. This was one of the personal experiences I shared with Phantom. I also let him know that I had to hustle because I had a fear that no one would hire me. I didn't know the power of God at the time.

Sometimes he made me feel like I had to worry about him not helping me if things didn't go his way. He got his way because I was scared. This went on for four years. The money was good, but I was not happy or satisfied. I wanted more, and I knew I could accomplish more. Eventually during that time I went from his work partner to his mistress. He not only gave me money to save, he took care of all my bills, my daughter, sent me on trips... I got whatever I wanted, no matter the cost. He did whatever it took to have me that way for as long as possible. Sounds like the life of a diva, but in reality it was a horrible experience. It was degrading and dishonest, and I wanted out.

It was a Tuesday night around 7pm, and I arrived at Bible study. I always made sure to listen and take in everything that was being said. The pastor told everyone to stand up. He said, "If there is a change you want to take place in your life, close your eyes and think about it." I closed my eyes and said to myself, *I want to gain my independence back and get away from Phantom.* The pastor then said, "Step out in faith and trust God."

A week later, Phantom and my friendship ended. I was out of work for almost two years. In the meantime, I lived off of my savings, went on food stamps, and decided to go back to school to finish my nursing degree. I changed my diet, attended the gym regularly, attended church every Tuesday, and decided to write my first book.

I was paying for school, a car note and insurance, utility bills, my business taxes, and I took care of myself and my daughter with the little that I had saved. After almost two years, my money began to run low. I decided I would have to get a job. When I was in my early twenties, I signed up to get a voucher I could use to get training in different fields. I received a $2500 voucher from a place called Work Force One. I followed all the rules and attended all the different sessions to receive the voucher. Later on, I decided to use my voucher at a driving school. It was a very small driving school, but comfortable. Through the driving school I gained my CDL driver's license. I was not interested in being a bus driver or driving any vans. But I figured it was a opportunity, and I took it. I had the license for a couple of years, but did not use it. But it did come in handy.

Once I realized that I needed a job, I phoned a childhood friend of mine who worked for a school bus company. I let her know that I had my CDL license and I needed a job. She contacted her boss, and I was told to meet with him a few days later. I had all my documents required to get the job, but I had to do a new road test, which I passed. But then one thing came up: my arrest for the fight I had with the girl. It was bittersweet news for me, because no other arrest was on my record. I was told that I had to go to the courthouse to get all my depositions. Surprisingly, that was the only one. I had been arrested in the past for shoplifting, but that did not come up. I was so happy to learn this information. The next thing I had to do was go with the deposition to the Board of Education and speak with someone about my case. I was nervous, but I had my faith to hold on to. This was an experience that I did not want to ever have to face again.

As I arrived at the Board of Education, I had to be scanned, and then I was told to go up to the fifth floor. Once I arrived, I let the receptionist know what I was there for. She told me to sign a paper and wait for my name to be called. While waiting, I thought about my life and how badly I wanted the job. I wanted to confirm how good God was, to feel normal, and to know I could get a good job just like anyone else. I was a changed woman and destined to do the right thing, desperate for opportunity.

I heard my name called by a heavyset Caucasian guy. He told me to have a seat at his desk. I handed him my deposition. he read it, then told me to go back to the bus company and tell them that Joe said clear, and that he would email them his paperwork by the following day. I looked at him, puzzled, and asked, "Do I get the job?"

He smiled and said, "Absolutely." I was so happy I could have hugged him, but I did not. I thanked him and went back to the bus company.

I arrived back at the bus company within about forty-five minutes. I gave them the message, and they gave me my ID card and my route. I left, stunned and teary eyed. I walked slowly to my car, reflecting on my past. I thought about all I been through. I thought about how I'd feared looking for a job. I thought about how real God was. Last but not least, I thought about how good it felt to do the right thing. I had tried every way possible to make it in life, and it had brought nothing but fear, heartache, and pain. I thanked God and said I was going to do it his way. I was going to be humble, pray, and be patient. I would trust God, put my fears behind me, and take back everything the devil had taken from me. That day I was not only a school bus driver, but I was back in school trying to finish my nursing degree. I was taking care of my aunt, who was suffering from Alzheimer's. Makayla was doing great as well. She was nine years old and loved to sing and bake things. I was very close with my family, attending church every Tuesday night for Bible study, and I was in the process of having my second baby girl.

Life might not have turned out how I wanted it to, but I was happier than I'd ever been. I made a lot of bad choices, which I faced the consequences for. I also made a lot of good choices in life, which allowed me to not only smile, but to be at peace within. I totally felt like the timing was right.

It's never too late to make a change and pursue your dreams. Writing a book was not in my plans, even though I always enjoyed writing and found comfort in doing it. I do plan to continue writing and am excited about publishing my second book, *From Lesbo To Prego.*